U0270138

PUBLIC HEALTH IN CHINA SERIES
Series Editor Liming Li

Infectious Disease in China
The Best Practical Cases

Editor   Wei-Zhong Yang

People's Medical Publishing House

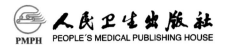

PMPH PEOPLE'S MEDICAL PUBLISHING HOUSE

Website: http://www.pmph.com/

Book Title: Infectious Disease in China: the Best Practical Cases
(Public Health in China Series)
中国公共卫生：重大疾病防治实践（英文版）

Contact address: No. 19, Pan Jia Yuan Nan Li, Chaoyang District, Beijing 100021, P.R. China, phone/fax: 8610 5978 7584, E-mail: pmph@pmph.com

First published: 2018
ISBN: 978-7-117-26001-5

Cataloguing in Publication Data:
A catalogue record for this book is available from the CIP-Database China.

Printed in The People's Republic of China

ISBN 978-7-117-26001-5

9 787117 260015>

Contributors

Tian Bai, MPH

Chinese National Influenza Center, National Institute for Viral Disease Control and Prevention, Chinese Center for Disease Control and Prevention
Beijing, China

Wu-Chun Cao, PhD

Department of Infectious Disease Epidemiology, Institute of Microbiology and Epidemiology, Beijing, China

Fu-Qiang Cui, MD, MPH, MPM, PhD

Professor and Head of Department of Laboratorial Science and Technology
Chair of Vaccine Research Center
School of Public Health, Peking University
Beijing, China

Li-Qun Fang, PhD

Department of Infectious Disease Epidemiology, Institute of Microbiology and Epidemiology, Beijing, China

Zhong-Jie Li, PhD

Deputy Director, Division of Infectious Disease, Key Laboratory of Surveillance and Early-warning on Infectious Disease, Chinese Center for Disease Control and Prevention
Beijing, China

Hui-Ming Luo, MD

Director, Department of Education and Training, Chinese Center for Disease Control and Prevention
Beijing, China

Ning Miao, MPH

Assistant Researcher, Division of Hepatitis, National Immunization Program (NIP), Chinese Center for Disease Control and Prevention

Beijing, China

Yue-Long Shu, PhD

Dean of Public Health School (Shenzhen), Sun Yat-sen University. Adjunct professor of National Institute for Viral Disease Control and Prevention, Chinese Center for Disease Control and Prevention

Beijing, China

Xiao-Jin Sun, MPH

Assistant Researcher, Division of Hepatitis, National Immunization Program (NIP), Chinese Center for Disease Control and Prevention

Beijing, China

Da-Yan Wang, PhD

Director of Chinese National Influenza Center, National Institute for Viral Disease Control and Prevention, Chinese Center for Disease Control and Prevention

Beijing, China

Fu-Zhen Wang, MPH

Deputy Director, Division of Hepatitis, National Immunization Program (NIP), Chinese Center for Disease Control and Prevention

Beijing, China

Li-Ping Wang, MD, PhD

Director, Branch of General Affairs on Infectious Disease, Division of Infectious Disease, Key Laboratory of Surveillance and Early-warning on Infectious Disease, Chinese Center for Disease Control and Prevention

Beijing, China

Xiao-Qi Wang, MSc

Director, Office of International Cooperation, Chinese Center for Disease Control and Prevention

Beijing, China

Ning Wen, MSc

National Immunization Program, Chinese Center for Disease Control and Prevention

Beijing, China

Dan Xiao, PhD

Department of Infectious Disease Epidemiology, Beijing Institute of Microbiology and Epidemiology

Beijing, China

Cui-Ling Xu, PhD

Chinese National Influenza Center, National Institute for Viral Disease Control and Prevention, Chinese Center for Disease Control and Prevention

Beijing, China

Wei-Zhong Yang, MD

Executive Vice-President & Secretary General, Chinese Preventive Medicine Association

Vice President of CAST UN Consultative Committee on Life Science & Human Health (CCLH)

Beijing, China

Wen-Wu Yin, M.D, MPH

Director, Branch of zoonotic and vector borned Infectious Disease, Division of Infectious Disease, Key Laboratory of Surveillance and Early-warning on Infectious Disease, Chinese Center for Disease Control and Prevention

Beijing, China

Guo-Min Zhang, PhD

Director, Division of Hepatitis, National Immunization Program (NIP), Chinese Center for Disease Control and Prevention

Beijing, China

Hui Zheng, MPH

Associate Researcher, Division of Hepatitis, National Immunization Program (NIP), Chinese Center for Disease Control and Prevention

Beijing, China

Ling-Qiao Zheng

Associate Senior Reporter for Chinese official health industry newspaper JianKangBao, Veteran reporter in the field of public health and infectious diseases prevention

Beijing, China

Wen- Fei Zhu, PhD

Chinese National Influenza Center, National Institute for Viral Disease Control and Prevention, Chinese Center for Disease Control and Prevention

Beijing, China

Reviewer

Xiao-Chen Dai, MSc, MPH, PhD

Department of Global Health

University of Washington

Washington, USA

Preface

Infectious diseases are borderless. China has made great achievements in infectious disease control and prevention in the past decades. The law on infectious diseases revised in 2004 acts as a powerful legal foundation to the national-wide surveillance and control of infectious disease. The national system, network and control strategies of infectious disease control have been optimized, and a web-based real-time reporting system has been put into use since 2004. The overall morbidity of infectious diseases has been relatively stable in recent years and showed a declining trend. Meanwhile, we have made and sustained effective response to the emerging disease outbreaks such as human streptococcus suis, influenza H1N1, influenza A (H7N9) et al, and to the re-emerging diseases such as tuberculosis, dengue fever, et al. The prevention and control of HIV/AIDS, TB and Hepatitis B, which constitute the major burden of infectious diseases in China, has made tremendous progress since 2003.

This book contains five stories of our battles against five specific diseases, namely, SARS, Influenza H1N1, Polio, Hepatitis B, and Human Streptococcus suis, Every story tells about how these infectious disease epidemics are solved, responses made to the outbreaks, and lessons learnt and experience gained, which are worth sharing and serve as the learning cases for public health professionals in other countries of the world.

Wei-Zhong Yang

Contents

Chapter 1

What have we learnt from SARS in mainland China

Wu-Chun Cao, Li-Qun Fang, and Dan Xiao

This chapter gives an overview of the severe acute respiratory syndrome (SARS) epidemic in mainland China and of what we have learnt since the outbreak. The epidemic spanned a large geographical extent but clustered in two regions: first in Guangdong Province, and about 3 months later in Beijing and its surrounding areas. The resulting case fatality ratio of 6.4% was less than half of that in other SARS-affected countries or regions, partly due to younger age of patients and higher proportion of community-acquired infections. Strong political commitment and a centrally coordinated response were most important for controlling SARS. The long-term economic consequence of the epidemic was limited. Many recovered patients suffer from avascular osteonecrosis, as a consequence of corticosteroid usage during their infection. The SARS epidemic provided valuable experience and lessons relevant in controlling outbreaks of emerging infectious diseases, and has led to fundamental reforms of the Chinese health system, and has substantially improved infrastructures, surveillance systems, and capacity to response to health emergencies. In particular, a comprehensive nationwide internet-based disease reporting system was established.

1.1　Introduction

In 2003, the world was confronted with the emergence of a new and in many cases fatal infectious disease, severe acute respiratory syndrome (SARS). The first case with typical symptoms of SARS emerged in Foshan municipality, Guangdong Province, China, with the onset date of 16 November 2002.[1] Five index cases were reported in

Foshan, Zhongshan, Jiangmen, Guangzhou and Shenzhen municipalities of Guang-dong Province before January 2003. The early-stage outbreak of SARS in Guangdong province was sporadic and apparently not associated with the index cases.[2] By January 2003, SARS had become a large-scale outbreak in Guangdong Province,[3] and after February 2003, it had appeared in Hong Kong[4] and seven other provinces including Guangxi, Jiangxi, Fujian, Hunan, Zhejiang, Sichuan and Shanxi.[5] Some cases from Shanxi Province and Hong Kong were imported to Beijing and transmission from index cases was amplified within several health care facilities by March.[6] Soon Beijing became the epicentre of SARS and endangered various other provinces or cities of mainland China. At the same time, Singapore, Canada, the United States of America and Vietnam were involved in the worldwide spread through imported cases from Hong Kong.[7] The World Health Organization (WHO) issued the first global alert on 12 March 2003 regarding a cluster of cases of severe atypical pneumonia in hospitals in Hong Kong, Hanoi and Guangdong.[8] Three days later, WHO issued an emergency travel advisory. On 24 March, WHO described the clinical features of SARS, which were revised on 1 May 2003[9] A novel coronavirus, named SARS-CoV, was identified as the infectious agent responsible for SARS in April 2003.[10,11] Soon thereafter, cases were reported from 32 countries and regions (later corrected to 29). In total, 8437 prob-able SARS cases, of whom 813 had died, were reported during the SARS epidemic of 2002-2003. Mainland China was the most seriously affected area, reporting 5327 prob-able SARS cases of whom 343 died, between 16 November 2002 and 11 June 2003.

As a result of initial lack of awareness of SARS by health workers, the disease spread unnoticed at the early stage of the epidemic, which was unduly prolonged by limited share of information. At the time, a functional infectious diseases surveil-lance system was not yet available, and the reporting system was outdated, hamper-ing data collection and delaying interventions. The SARS outbreak brought China virtually to a standstill, forcing the country to thoroughly review its infectious dis-ease control policies. Since then, the Chinese government has implemented new and innovative strategies, strengthened the constructions of the relevant legal system and the disease prevention and control system, and made huge investments to improve infrastructures, surveillance systems, and emergency preparedness and response capacity, such as a real-time monitoring system that is now serving as a model for worldwide surveillance and response to infectious disease threats.[12] The world has moved on since the SARS epidemic, but the insights gained in mainland China remain valuable, with comparable infectious disease threats presenting continuously.

1.2　Description of the epidemic

During the 2002−2003 SARS outbreak, mainland China reported 5327 probable cases, of whom 343 died, giving a case fatality ratio (CFR) of 6.4%. The epidemic spanned a large geographical extent (170 counties of 22 provinces) but clustered in two areas: first in Guangdong Province, and about 3 months later in Beijing with its surrounding areas Shanxi, Inner Mongolia Autonomic Region, Hebei and Tianjin. Figure 1.1 shows the temporal distribution of SARS in the six most seriously affected geographic areas of mainland China. Spatiotemporal analyses indicated that the spread of SARS occurred in two different patterns.[13] In the early stage of the epidemic, especially before strict control measures were taken, SARS spread to new areas randomly through certain index cases. Thereafter, human travel along transportation routes influenced the transmission of SARS, as illustrated by the spread of SARS in Middle-north China and South China. The epidemic period in middle-north China was shorter than in South China, but the geographic spread was wider. SARS not only spread locally, but also diffused quickly and resulted in several outbreaks in areas of middle-north China close to Beijing city. In contrast, the SARS epidemic in South China was mainly limited to Guangdong Province.

　　Transportation routes accelerated the spread of SARS in mainland China. However, national highways and inter-provincial freeways appeared to play a critical role (Figure 1.2), whereas railways seemed to be less important.[13]

　　For the definition of SARS cases a distinction was made between probable and suspected cases on the basis of contact history and the number and severity of symptoms. In China, it was only possible late in the epidemic to confirm SARS through serological tests. In a study comparing clinical characteristics of probable and suspected cases it was found that although symptoms hardly differed, there were clearly different haematological profiles, justifying the distinction between probable and suspected cases and confirming that the suspected cases most likely did not have SARS.[14]

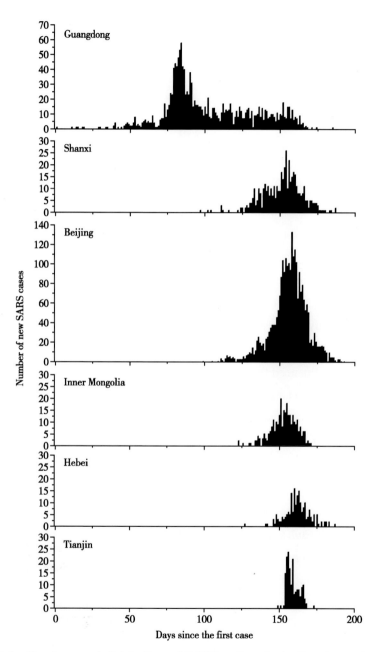

Figure 1.1 The temporal distribution of SARS outbreaks in the six most seriously affected geographic areas of mainland China by plotting the number of new cases per day of onset since the first SARS case on November 16, 2002, in Guangdong Province.

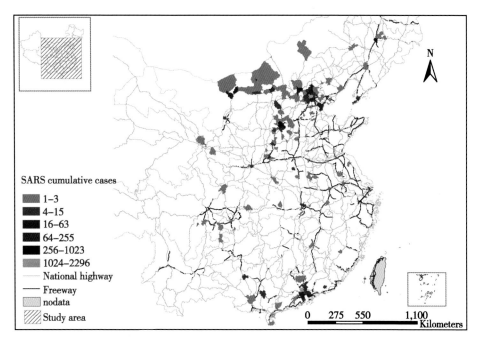

Figure 1.2   The cumulative incidence map of the SARS epidemic in mainland China, overlapping national highway and inter-provincial freeway maps. Cumulative cases are indicated by coloured gradients and indicate the number of cases per county/township.

The average duration (3.8 days) and pattern (with time of epidemic and age) of onset of symptoms to hospital admission of SARS patients in mainland China were comparable to other affected areas.[15] The duration of hospital admission to discharge for those who survived (29.7 days) was shorter than elsewhere in the world, possibly because of different hospitalisation policies. The duration of hospital admission to death in mainland China was 17.4 days, which is also shorter than in other areas.

In the course of time, hospital epidemics in particular were rapidly brought under control, with increasing efficiency.[16] This was due to increasing understanding of the disease and more effective preventive measures such as establishing isolation wards, training and monitoring hospital staff in infection control, screening of health care workers (HCWs), and compliance with the use of personal protection equipment.[17]

1.3   Case fatality

Figure 1.3 compares the CFRs for SARS patients of different ages in Beijing, Guangdong and Tianjin. Because of their deteriorated health status and apparent complications, the mortality rate increased significantly among patients aged 50 and above. The Tianjin SARS outbreak happened mainly within hospitals, leading to a high impact of co-morbidity, which explains the relatively high CFR. Guangdong Province showed a considerably lower CFR than Beijing, the reason of which is still unclear. The overall CFR in mainland China was 6.4% which was much lower than that reported in other areas and countries (Table 1.1), where CFRs varied from 9.7% in Vietnam to 17.2% in Hong Kong. The much lower case fatality in mainland China was also in contrast with the shorter duration of hospital admission to death compared to other countries or regions. The obvious reasons for the lower CFR are young age of the patients and a relatively higher number of community acquired infections as opposed to hospital acquired infections. However, the relatively young age of the cases (median age 33 years) only partly (approximately 25%) explains the low CFR in mainland China compared to other affected countries and areas, where patients' median age varied from 37 years in Singapore to 49 years in Canada (Table 1.1). [18] The relatively lower proportion of hospital acquired infections in mainland China – reflected in the lower proportion of infections among HCW compared to other areas (19% vs. 23 – 56%; see Table 1.1) – is also only partly responsible for the lower CFR in mainland China, especially since this factor is highly correlated with age.

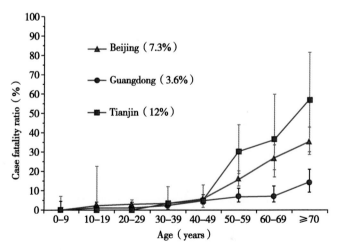

Figure 1.3 Comparison of the case fatality ratios of different ages for SARS patients in Beijing, Guangdong and Tianjin. Intervals indicate 90% binomially distributed confidence intervals. The values in parentheses represent the overall case fatality ratio for each area.

Table 1.1   The characteristics of SARS outbreak in mainland China and
in other countries or regions

Country or area	Mainland China	Hong Kong	Taiwan	Singa-pore	Vietnam	Canada
Number of cases	5327	1755	674	238	62	251
CFR: no. dead (%)	343 (6.4)	302 (17.2)	87 (12.9)	33 (13.9)	6 (9.7)	43 (17.1)
Age: median (yrs)	33	40	46	37	43	49
Occupation: HCW (%)	1021 (19.2)	405 (23.1)	205 (30.3)	97 (40.8)	35 (56.5)	101 (40.2)

It has been suggested that mainland China had a substantial number of cases that were not really SARS, especially in Guangdong, where the epidemic started. A review study comparing seroprevalence rates in different SARS affected areas did show relatively lower seroprevalence in mainland China, but the differences in other areas were only small and far from significant. However, even if the lower seroprevalence that was found in mainland China actually represented over-reporting, then this factor could only explain a modest 10% of the lower case fatality.[19] Thus, there still remains a challenge in explaining the lower death rates in mainland China. It may be due to better treatment (see below) and use of Chinese traditional medicines.

1.4   The effect of interventions

During the SARS epidemic in mainland China, various interventions were implemented to contain the outbreak.[20] Overall speaking, the measures taken were certainly effective, given the fact that the epidemic was fully controlled within 200 days after the first case emerged. The method of Wallinga and Teunis,[21] with quantifications from Lipsitch et al,[22] was used to estimate R_t, the effective or net reproduction number, which helps to determine which interventions were most important. R_t is defined as the mean number of secondary cases infected by one primary case with symptom onset on day t. This number changes during the course of an epidemic, particularly as a result of effective control measures. If R_t is larger than the threshold value of one, a sustained chain of transmission will occur, eventually leading to a major epidemic. If this number is maintained below one, then transmission may still continue, but the number of secondary cases is not sufficient to replace the primary cases, leading to a gradual fade-out of the epidemic.

Figure 1.4 shows R_t over time for mainland China along with the timing of nine important events and public health control measures. The graph is characterised by a fluctuating pattern and wide confidence interval early in the epidemic, which can be explained by the initial low number of cases used in the calculations and the relatively more important impact of so-called 'super-spreading events'. In Guangdong, where the epidemic started, standard control measures such as isolation and contact tracing (arrow 2) seem to already have helped to largely interrupt transmission in this province. However, during the period from day 80 to 140 the number of new SARS cases steadily increased, due to the spread to and within other parts of China, i.e. mainly Beijing and its surrounding provinces. The first official report of an outbreak in Guangdong (arrow 3) and the WHO global alerts (arrow 4) were by no means reflected in a consistent reduction of R_t. Also, the first interventions in Beijing were not effective enough to cause any downward trend in the transmission (arrow 5). It was only around 11-14 April 2003 that the Chinese authorities gained full control of all activities to combat SARS, with national, unambiguous, rational, widely followed guidelines and control measures, under central guidance (arrow 6). Immediately the reproduction number decreased dramatically and consistently. Within one week, R_t was below one. Strikingly, this marked decrease after the period 11-14 April was consistently present in the patterns of R_t for all heavily affected areas in mainland China.[23] The stringent control measures to prevent human contacts (arrow 7), including the decision to cancel the public holiday of May 1 (arrow 8), were all initiated after R_t was below one, i.e. when the epidemic was already dying off, again consistently for all areas in mainland China. Given the information available at the time, the most stringent interventions were rational since it was not clear to which extent the epidemic was under control. However, looking retrospectively, we can now conclude that these measures – which severely affected public life – contributed little to the factual containment of the SARS epidemic; the essential moment had occurred earlier. That being said, the late interventions may still have played a role in speeding up the elimination of SARS. Also, cancelling the public holiday, when millions of people travel long distances to visit their family, may have prevented (smaller) outbreaks in yet unaffected locations.

We conclude that strong political commitment and a centrally coordinated response was the most important factor in the control of SARS in mainland China. With respect to future outbreaks of emerging infectious diseases, we emphasise that it is of first and foremost importance that effective control is based on clear (inter) national guidelines, communication and reporting structures, along with firm determination and responsibilities at all levels.

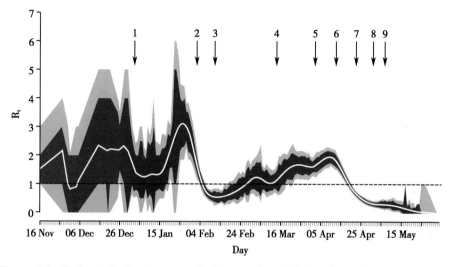

Figure 1.4 Estimated effective reproduction number (Rt) (number of secondary infections generated per primary case) during the SARS epidemic in China. Values represent average Rt (central white line) and associated 95% (grey) and 80% (black) confidence intervals, by date of symptom onset. The critical value of Rt = 1, below which sustained transmission is impossible, is marked with a broken horizontal line. Arrows reflect the time of important events and public health control measures: (1) Local newspaper report about outbreak of unknown infectious disease in Guangdong (2 January); (2) Start of control in Guangdong hospitals: e.g. isolation, contact tracing (1 - 3 February); (3) First official report of outbreak by Guangdong authorities (11 February); (4) WHO global alerts; first mentioning of SARS (12 - 15 March); (5) First protocol of SARS control; start isolation in Beijing hospitals (2 April); (6) Mandatory reporting of SARS; definition of diagnostic criteria and treatment (11 - 14 April); (7) Stringent control measures: quarantine in airports and stations; closure of schools, universities and public places; daily reporting by the national media (19 - 26 April); (8) Public holiday cancelled; new 1000-bed SARS hospital opened (1 May); (9) Further improvement of various guidelines and protocols (4 - 9 May).

1.5   Consequences of the epidemic

There were many obvious immediate consequences of the epidemic, such as substantial morbidity and mortality, fear for becoming infected, panic in the public domain, stringent quarantine measures, travel restrictions, etc. In addition, two important middle and long-term consequences of the epidemic were identified. First, there was the economic impact. This was studied for Beijing by Beutels *et al.*[24] through associating time series of daily and monthly SARS cases and deaths and volume of public train, airplane and cargo transport, tourism, household consumption patterns and gross domestic product growth in Beijing. The authors concluded that leisure activities, local and international transport and tourism were severely affected by SARS, particularly in May 2003. Much of this consumption was merely postponed; but irrecoverable losses to the tourism alone were estimated at about US$ 1.4 billion, or 300 times the cost of treatment for SARS cases in Beijing.

Second, there were long-term health consequences for the SARS patients who were treated with corticosteroids. Lv *et al.* investigated the relationship between avascular osteonecrosis (AVN) and corticosteroid treatment given to SARS patients through a longitudinal study of 71 SARS patients (mainly HCWs) who had been treated with corticosteroids, with an observation time of 36 months.[25] Magnetic resonance images and X-rays of hips, knees, shoulders, ankles and wrists were taken as part of the post-SARS follow-up assessments. Thirty-nine per cent developed AVN of the hips within 3-4 months after starting treatment. Two more cases of hip necrosis were seen after 1 year and another 11 cases of AVN were diagnosed after 3 years, one with hip necrosis and 10 with necrosis in other joints. In total, a staggering 58% of the cohort had developed AVN after 3 years of observation. The sole factor explaining AVN in the hip was the total dose of corticosteroids received. The use of corticosteroids has been debated, with conflicting opinions about steroids being the key component in the treatment of SARS.[26] It has remained uncertain whether the aggressive use of corticosteroids during the SARS epidemic has tipped the balance. Has the use of high dose corticosteroids saved more lives and been responsible for the lower case fatality in mainland China? And, do immediate benefits in terms of saving lives outweigh the adverse effects, including AVN?

1.6   Lessons learnt and actions taken in China regarding epidemic preparedness

The SARS epidemic provided valuable experience and lessons relevant to controlling outbreaks of newly emerging infectious diseases, which are surely due to come. Human infection with avian influenza viruses, the novel A (H1N1) influenza, and imported infectious diseases such as the Zika virus disease and yellow fever disease are already knocking at our doors! Important lessons learnt in China included the need for more honesty and transparency, improvement of surveillance, laboratory facilities and case management.[27] Also, public health measures to control infectious diseases, reporting systems, and central guidance and coordination came under scrutiny. Another lesson was the need to inform and involve the public timely and adequately regarding control measures. There was a strong realisation that the best defence against any threat of newly emerging infectious diseases is a robust public health system in its science, capacity, practice, and through collaboration with clinical and veterinary medicine, academia, industry, and other public and private partners.

An important resolution of the Chinese government was to improve its disease surveillance system to rapidly identify newly emerging infectious diseases and to minimise their spread in China and to the rest of the world. The traditional surveillance network using reporting cards filled out by hand and sent by mail or fax has been substituted by an automatic information system called the China Information System for Disease Control and Prevention (CISDCP), which is the world's largest internet-based disease reporting system.[12] The government has also increased their investment into enhancing the capabilities of detecting, diagnosing, preventing and controlling of newly emerging infectious diseases at various levels. New and innovative strategies have been established for response to health emergencies, such as the establishment of the parallel laboratory confirmation mechanism for newly emerging infectious pathogens to reduce the risk of errors, rapid disclosure of information to the WHO and to the public, international information exchange and collaboration, as well as more information on public health and on infectious diseases to the public. What's more, the Chinese government has strengthened the relevant legal system and the disease prevention and control system, e.g., the revision of Law of People's Republic of China on the Prevention and Treatment of Infectious Disease in 2004, and the issue and implement of Regulations on Preparedness for and Response to Emergent Public Health Hazards in 2003, as well as the construction of the Chinese Centre for Disease Control and Prevention, and the improvements of surveillance systems of infectious diseases and preparedness and response capacity for emerging public health events.[28,29,30] Education and training projects such as training courses for public health officials and health care workers have been initiated, and new training has been added to the education programs of universities. Funds for research projects on the development of vaccines, drugs and diagnostic techniques have been granted to develop new approaches in the prevention, diagnosis and treatment of emerging infectious diseases.

In conclusion, the epidemic of a new infectious disease, SARS, took firstly China and subsequently many other areas in the world completely by surprise. Fortunately, the consequences of this epidemic in terms of people afflicted and economic loss were not entirely catastrophic. Also, it turned out that SARS could be controlled relatively easily through standard interventions. However, the epidemic revealed some important weaknesses in the Chinese public health system, which has been dealt with efficiently and successfully by the Chinese government. At the moment, China is better prepared than ever for epidemics, which may be much worse than SARS in terms of speed of spread and fatality rate. As a matter of fact, SARS can be seen just as a wake-up call.

References

1. Zhong NS, Zeng GQ. Management and prevention of SARS in China. In: SARS: A Case Study in Emerging Infections. Oxford University Press, Oxford, 2005, pp. 31-4.

2. He JF, Xu RH, Yu DW, et al. Severe acute respiratory syndrome in Guangdong Province of China: epidemiology and control measures. Zhonghua Yu Fang Yi Xue Za Zhi. 2003; 37,227-32.

3. Zhao Z, Zhang F, Xu M, et al. Description and clinical treatment of an early outbreak of severe

Southern California in the United States,[1] additional cases were rapidly reported from Texas, Chicago, Arizona, and New York. Then the virus spread rapidly to other nations. The World Health Organization (WHO) systematically applied the previously developed pandemic phases based on the extent of spread and declared a "public health emergency of international concern" on 25 April 2009. The alert level was immediately raised to phase 5, with the continuous spread reported in countries of North America. On 11 June 2009, the virus arrived in European countries, WHO raised the level of influenza A(H1N1) pandemic alert to phase 6. One year later, WHO officially declared that the pandemic is over on August 10, 2010. Afterwards, the pandemic H1N1 2009 virus co-circulates with H3N2 and B influenza viruses seasonally.

2.2 The responses to the pandemic H1N1 2009 in China

The first human case of H1N1 2009 in China was detected by Chengdu Center for Disease Control and Prevention (Chengdu CDC), and then confirmed by Sichuan provincial CDC and Chinese Center for Disease Control and Prevention (China CDC). This was an imported case from the United States. Very soon, more cases were reported from different provinces in China, accumulating to more than 120,000 human cases with 800 deaths by the end of the pandemic. It was estimated that 207.7 million individuals (15.9%) experienced pH1N1 infection in China based on a national wide cross-sectional sero-prevalence study.[2]

When WHO announced that A (H1N1) outbreak (named swine flu at the early stage) in Mexico and the United States was an "international public health concern" on April 25th, 2009, the emergency response actions were triggered immediately in China. Under the leadership of the State Council, a joint emergency response mechanism was established immediately. All 33 ministries were involved in a coordination body to fight against the 2009 pandemic. The Ministry of Health acted as the leader to communicate and cooperate with other departments according to their functions and responsibilities, and convened regular meetings to ensure the responses timely and effectively. A scientific advisory committee was also established under the joint response mechanism. This special scientific advisory committee provided technical support for evidence-based strategies and policy development. The joint emergency response system features unified command, graded responsibility, and is coordinated, orderly, and highly efficient. The goals for the pandemic response were to confine the epidemic and protect the public from security threats, to guarantee normal economic activities and to protect social harmony and stability.

2.2.1   Science-based strategies development with timely update based on different epidemic situations

China developed the pandemic preparedness and response plan after the first H5N1 human infection was reported in 2005. Strategies including surveillance, laboratories capacity building, vaccine development and stockpiling have been developed. However, it was the first time for China to respond to the influenza pandemic after SARS outbreak in 2003, there existed great challenges and much pressures. With the guidance of expert consultant committee, the strategies for prevention and control were developed with timely updates based on new evidence and epidemic situations.

The whole response procedure could be divided into two major steps including the early containment phase and late mitigation phase. The strategy was to stringently prevent the imported case before the first confirmed human case was reported. The activities included strengthening the exit-entry inspection and quarantine, enhancing surveillance, conducting communication and education campaign, and carrying out research on diagnostic reagents, antiviral drugs and vaccine. After the first human case was reported on 11 May 2009, the surveillance network expanded, and many hospitals were designated for influenza patient treatment and the infection control in these hospitals was further enhanced.

The strategy was adjusted to reduce domestic transmission, prevent community outbreak and to improve the treatment of severe cases after the WHO announced the pandemic on 11 June 2009. The activities included improving port inspection and quarantine measures, strengthening prevention and control work in schools and communities and expediting vaccine clinical trials.

The strategy was adjusted again to reduce the impact of outbreak and to minimize the morbidity and mortality of the disease if the pandemic influenza virus spread in China widely. The activities included improving the clinical treatment especially for the severe cases, vaccination in high-risk groups and enhancing the risk communication and health promotion.

2.2.2 Diagnostic kits development and laboratory surveillance capacity building (Figure 2.2)

Patient diagnosis was crucial for pandemic response, it was the first step to provide treatment to patients, to quarantine patients and monitor their close contacts. CNIC developed the diagnostic kits successfully within 72 hours after the US Centers for Disease Control and Prevention (CDC) provided the pandemic H1N1 virus and sequences. The diagnostic kits were distributed to all national influenza surveillance network, quarantine and inspection laboratories and other 13 countries such as Cuba, Mongolia and ASEAN countries. The influenza surveillance network expanded from 63 laboratories to 411 laboratories in order to strengthen the diagnostic capacity in China. This network played an important role for patient treatment and epidemic control and prevention; almost all of the confirmed human cases were diagnosed through this network. What' more, this network was also essential to monitor the virus mutation and provide scientific evidences for risk assessment. At the early stage, the data for hospitalizations and deaths demonstrated big differences among different countries, cases in Mexico appeared to be more severe than those in the United States. In addition, people worried that the virus could mutate to become more virulent like 1918 Spanish pandemic H1N1 virus; thus it was very important to monitor the virus mutations and evolutions timely. More than 1000 pandemic H1N1 viruses had been sequenced, and the sequence data demonstrated that the viruses circulated in China had no difference from those circulated in other countries, and carried no known genetic markers associated with increased disease severity. Timely genetic sequencing data were also instrumental to monitor the antiviral drugs resistance, provided the evidence for the clinical treatment, helped to identify the emergence of new mutations associated with more severe outcomes, and tracked any changes that might represent an increasing drift from chosen vaccine viruses. All these data supported the technical guidance development and update.

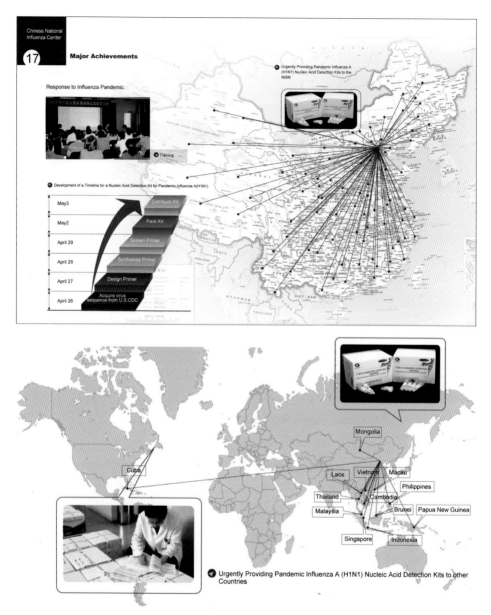

Figure 2.2   Timely development and distribution of diagnostic kit for pandemic H1N1 2009.

2.2.3   Enhanced exit-entry point inspection and quarantine, and stringent close contacts monitoring at the early stage

All people entering China are required to fill in the health declaration form at the port of entry, all suspected cases with influenza like illness would be transferred to the designated hospitals for quarantine and treatment; if the specimen collected from the patients are tested positive, their close contacts will be monitored for 7 days called "medical observation". The effectiveness of border screening is still controversial. Some studies showed that border screening could only postpone the spread of pandemic virus by a few days, while other studies indicated the border screening and quarantine delayed the outbreak peak for at least a few month, there were two peaks in May and October respectively in the US, but only one peak occurred in October in China.

2.2.4　Promote vaccine development and vaccination campaign

Vaccination is the most important measure for the pandemic prevention and control, however, the seasonal influenza vaccine could not provide cross protection due to the antigenic drift between pandemic H1N1 2009 and seasonal H1N1, thus successful development of a new vaccine was in urgent need. The Ministry of Health of China coordinated all efforts for pandemic H1N1 vaccine development under a joint coordination mechanism. Ten departments including National Development and Reform Commission, the Ministry of Health, Ministry and Information Technology, State Food and Drug Administration, China CDC, China Pharmaceutical and Biological Products Office and ten influenza vaccine production enterprises were actively engaged. This world's biggest clinical trial recruited 12,691 volunteers in ten centers and was conducted in China only one month after the pandemic was announced (Figure 2.3).[3] The clinical data demonstrated that the A (H1N1) vaccine has similar safety and immunogenicity results as the seasonal influenza vaccine. One dose of non-adjuvant split-virion vaccine containing 7.5 microg haemagglutinin could be promoted as the formulation of choice against 2009 pandemic influenza A H1N1 for people aged 12 years and above. In children (aged <12 years), two 7.5 microg doses might be needed. Eventually, the 15 microg non-adjuvant split vaccine was approved by the State Food and Drug Administration in early September, making China the world's first country to complete vaccine development and registration successfully. The related clinical data also revised the recommendation by WHO that at least two doses of pandemic vaccines were needed to provide protection. The mass vaccination campaign started immediately. By 14 April 2010, 151.5 million doses of vaccines had been released by SFDA, and 97.2 million people, representing 7.3% of the population, had been vaccinated against the H1N1 virus. The vaccination efficacy was estimated to be 87%. The detailed side effect information was collected from 89.6 million vaccinated participants through the National Adverse Events Following Immunization (AEFI) Surveillance System, which was established in 2005. The results demonstrated that the pattern of adverse events was similar to those with seasonal influenza vaccines; there was no evidence of an increased risk of the Guillain–Barré syndrome, which was rare but was found to be associated with a vaccine against the "swine flu" virus during the 1976–1977 in the United States. Therefore, the AEFI surveillance data are of great significance to evaluate the safety of a new pandemic H1N1 vaccine.

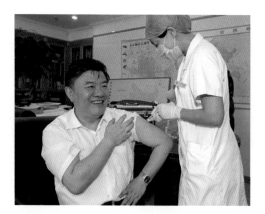

Figure 2.3   Chen Zhu, the former health minister, received the pandemic H1N1 vaccine in the trial.

2.2.5   Improve the treatment of patients

Clinical treatment in the healthcare system, with enhanced surge capacity, is one of the most important responses to mitigate the pandemic's impact. Clinic case management and treatment guideline was rapidly developed and updated timely, and available to all health sectors. In the containment phase, a limited number of imported cases were detected. To slow down the spread of the disease, all patients with confirmed infection were treated in the designated hospitals despite the fact that the majority had mild illness. Antivirals were distributed into the designated hospitals from the national and local stockpiles, and were used to treat the confirmed or clinically diagnosed H1N1 cases. Antivirals were also provided to high-risk close contacts, including pregnant women, persons with severe chronic medical conditions, children aged <5 years, elderly people aged 65 years and above, and healthcare workers. During the initial 2 months, 82.3% of confirmed H1N1 mild cases were administered oseltamivir (72.4% within 48 hours of the onset of illness).

Since July, when the mitigation phase started, China focused on managing and treating patients with severe illness. Antiviral drugs production and distribution were accelerated to prepare for the pandemic's peak. Patients were treated in designated hospitals to make optimal use of healthcare resources. Antivirals were recommended to those with severe or high-risk infections. In addition, the Chinese government strengthened the treatment capacity of low-income provinces through additional investments in medical facilities and stockpiles.

With the extensive H1N1 infections, there was a sharp increase in the number of people seeking for health services. Outpatient attendance peaked in October 2009, and the outpatient and emergency services of healthcare system were overwhelmed, especially in many major cities in the Northern provinces. To cope with the increased demand for emergency and critical care services, the Ministry of Health mobilized surge capacity by training doctors, increasing the number of designated hospitals and back-up hospitals, triaging and prioritizing services to manage the surge in case numbers, and establishing counterpart support mechanisms between provinces and hospitals. These responses optimized treatment with limited resources, and played a key role in decreasing the number of deaths caused by H1N1 infection.

2.2.6 Traditional Chinese medicine usage

Other treatments, such as traditional Chinese medicine and antiserum therapy, were also introduced. A prospective non-blinded, randomized and controlled clinical trial (Clinical Trials.gov registration number: NCT00935194) was conducted in 11 hospitals from 4 provinces in China.[4] A total of 410 laboratory-confirmed pdmH1N1 patients (aged 15 to 69 years) were included in this trial. The antiviral effect of Chinese traditional therapy maxingshigan-yinqiaosan was compared with oseltamivir.

The results showed that oseltamivir and maxingshigan-yinqiaosan, alone and in combination, reduced time to fever resolution in patients with pdmH1N1 influenza virus infection. These data suggest that maxingshigan-yinqiaosan may be used as an alternative treatment to H1N1 influenza virus infection. In this case, the use of traditional Chinese medicine was recommended in the Chinese guidelines for the treatment of H1N1 infection.

2.2.7　Strengthen the risk communication and health education

China considered the active communication with media as one of the most important measures for pandemic response. Public information and risk communication messages were disseminated through a variety of media, including television, radio, and extensively distributed printed materials. China set up a regular mechanism to timely release epidemic information and prevention and control progress, and established a 24/7 hotline 12320 taking enquiries. More importantly, it is very useful to monitor public opinions and to make real-time analysis and adjust media policy in time. These measures played an important role in maintaining the public social harmony and stability.

2.2.8　Strengthen the international cooperation

China convened a series of meetings with international organizations and countries since May 2009, including WHO, the US CDC, Public Health Agency of Canada, et al, to share the detailed information about the local epidemic situations and response measures. China obtained the pandemic A (H1N1) 2009 virus strain timely from the US, Canada and Hong Kong SAR, to support the development of laboratory testing kits and vaccine. At the same time, we dispatched personnel abroad to receive training about pandemic A (H1N1) 2009 surveillance. China CDC also organized training courses for ASEAN countries to share our technologies and experience.

　　The updated pandemic information in China was shared routinely to WHO, APEC, European Union, ASEAN, the United States, Mexico, Canada, Cuba, Japan, Korea et al., which enhanced the collaboration with and trust in China from international society.

2.3   Experience and lessons learned

2.3.1   An influenza pandemic can arise anywhere in the world and can emerge in any season

Before the 2009 pandemic occurred, people assumed that Southeast Asia might be the epicenter of influenza pandemics. This hypothesis was supported by the 1957 Asian H2N2 and the 1968 Hong Kong H3N2 pandemics. The high density of aquatic birds (ducks, geese), swine, and humans and live poultry markets in this region further supported this hypothesis. However, the Pandemic H1N1 2009 originating from Mexico indicates that pandemic influenza can emerge anywhere in the world. The precursors of the 2009 H1N1 pandemic virus were the triple reassortants from the United States, which had reassorted with the avian H1N1 viruses that adapted to pigs in Europe prior to 1979.

Influenza occurs in the winter season in temperate areas whereas in the tropics influenza occurs year round. However, the pandemic can occur any time, the Asian H2N2 1957 pandemic was first detected in February 1957 in Guizhou of southern China, whereas the Hong Kong H3N2 pandemic was first detected in Hong Kong in July 1968. The pandemic H1N1 2009 was first detected in humans in April 2009 but the earliest cases probably occurred in February 2009. The lesson learned is that the pandemics of influenza can arise anywhere and anytime, therefore, the global surveillance should be conducted yearly around the world.

2.3.2   A functional and high quality surveillance system is the foundation for epidemic response.

China established influenza surveillance in 2000. The system originally consisted of 8 network laboratories and 31 sentinel hospitals that reported ILI cases and isolated viruses for vaccine strain recommendation. By 2005, the system had expanded to 63 network laboratories and 197 sentinel hospitals in 31 provinces. In 2009, in response to the pandemic, the system further expanded to 411 laboratories and 556 hospitals, which covered all prefectures/cities and priority counties throughout the country

(Figure 2.4). During the last 10 years, more than 95% laboratories can perform real-time PCR detection, which makes the clinical diagnosis data available in the surveillance system. In addition, more than 70% of laboratories can perform virus isolation, and the virus isolates can be sent to CNIC for further characterizations such as genetic sequencing and antigenic analysis to provide timely evidences for risk assessment. This surveillance system can also detect any influenza virus with pandemic potential, such as recently discovered avian H7N9 influenza virus in China.

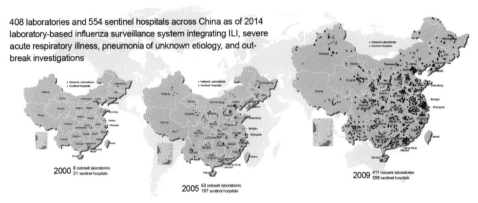

Figure 2.4   The expanded influenza surveillance networks in China after in pandemic H1N1 2009.

2.3.3   Joint emergency response mechanism and graded prevention strategy are the key to the scientific and efficient response

A joint prevention and control working mechanism led by the Ministry of Health and joined by 33 departments is the core of overall responses to H1N1 pandemic 2009, especially for the vaccine preparation and trials. This mechanism ensured that a strong command and control structure was established before the pandemic H1N1 virus spread to China, that an integrated approach was developed to coordinate actions taken by 33 different ministries, and that information sharing and risk communication were managed in a timely and accurate manner. In order to solve the bottleneck problems during the pandemic vaccine development, a "special mechanism that coordinated the R&D, registration and production of pandemic H1N1 vaccine" was established by the joint emergency response mechanism. With this mechanism, it only took 2 months to complete the clinical trial with around 13,000 volunteers, and to finish the vaccination campaign during the pandemic response.

China adopted a graded prevention strategy along with the development of the pandemic. This includes early containment phase and late mitigation phase. The early strategy was to stringently prevent the imported case and strategy shifted to late mitigation phase when it started to spread in China. At the early stage, all patients received isolation therapy, but it applied to only severe cases when response level was advanced to mitigation phase.

2.4 Conclusion

Pandemic H1N1 2009 was the first pandemic in the 21st century but will definitely not be the last one. Fortunately, this pandemic was moderate in severity. However, it was estimated that there were 201,200 respiratory deaths (range 105,700-395,600) and additional 83,300 cardiovascular deaths (46,000-179,900) were associated with pandemic influenza A(H1N1) 2009. Eighty percent of respiratory and cardiovascular deaths occurred in people less than 65 years old.

Nowadays, we are facing more challenges than ever before; the world is getting more crowded, connected and converged. The global population has been increasing exponentially and may reach 11 billion by the end of 2050 based on the current growth rate. To keep pace with the growing population, we need more poultry and pigs to provide enough proteins for life. Over the past 40 years, the amount of protein from poultry meat has increased by 3.4 times. For pig meat, it has increased by 1.6 times. The world is also getting more connected, a person can travel to anywhere in the world within an incubation time of influenza.

These rapidly changing situations require more extensive global cooperation and response. In addition, the prevention and control of influenza is impossible without ongoing monitoring of human and animal influenza viruses. One of the most important legacies from 2009 pandemic response is the expanded national influenza surveillance network in China. It is critical for this network to detect any pandemic potential influenza virus quickly, as it has demonstrated during H7N9 avian influenza outbreak response in 2013. Finally, the joint emergency response mechanisms set up at both national and international levels play such a vital role in curbing the influenza virus with pandemic potential.

References

1. Swine influenza A (H1N1) infection in two children--Southern California, March-April 2009. MMWR Morb Mortal Wkly Rep 2009; 58: 400-402.

2. Xu C, Bai T, Iuliano AD, et al. The seroprevalence of pandemic influenza H1N1 (2009) virus in China. PLoS One 2011;6(4).

3. Liang, X. F. et al. Safety and immunogenicity of 2009 pandemic influenza A H1N1 vaccines in China: a multicentre, double-blind, randomised, placebo-controlled trial. Lancet 2010; 375: 56-66.

4. Wang, C. et al. Oseltamivir compared with the Chinese traditional therapy maxingshigan-yinqiaosan in the treatment of H1N1 influenza: a randomized trial. Ann Intern Med 2011; 155:217-225.

Chapter 3

A War Against Polio Again - Blocking the Virus Ten Years After Polio Free

Hui-Ming Luo, Ning Wen, Wei-Zhong Yang

The last case of wild polio in China occurred in 1994. WHO Western Pacific Region, where China is located, achieved the goal of polio free in 2000, and maintained polio free status ever since. Unexpectedly, one outbreak of type 1 wild poliovirus (WPV1) was detected in Hotan in Southern Xinjiang Uygur Autonomous Region (Southern Xinjiang) in China with a total of 21 cases reported from 4 prefectures in July 2011.[1] The cases were confirmed to have been caused by WPV1 imported from Pakistan.

After detecting the outbreak, China initiated a level 2 public health emergency response promptly and carried out a series of response actions, including retrospective reviews and investigation of acute flaccid paralysis (AFP) cases, rapid assessment for vaccination coverage, initiation of daily Zero case reporting, immediate expansion of standard case definition and reporting sites, risk assessment, as well as 5 rounds of emergency immunization and supplementary immunization activities (SIAs). Under the support of international organizations and governments of all provinces, it took one and a half months for the government of Xinjiang to stop the outbreak and the last polio case was reported on October 9, 2011. WHO removed China from the list of polio endemic countries on April 10, 2012, China became polio free again.

The control of this outbreak set up a model that mobilized Chinese public health resources, coordinated among multiple ministries, and cooperated among social sources. After the outbreak was confirmed, all preparation work for polio vaccine SIAs was completed within 15 days. Looking back, the control process was thrilling but orderly. Governments of Xinjiang and other provinces, the Ministry of Health (MoH) and other relevant ministries was united and cooperated closely, with each partner fulfilling its own duty. The Ministry of Finance (MoF) and the Xinjiang government each appropriated 160 million Yuan in response to the outbreak. MoH deployed a total of 500 experts to Xinjiang, with 5 rounds of SIAs carried out and 43.63 million doses of vaccines used. Of the SIAs, 4 rounds in southern Xinjiang targeted persons aged up to 40 years old. MoH, Ministry of Education (MoE), Quality Inspection Administration, State Food and Drug Administration (SFDA), China National Biotechnology Group (CNBG), China Academy of Medical Sciences cooperated closely in the outbreak control process. Other departments, such as Ministry of Railways, air force, civil aviation bureau, provided strong supports. The strategies for outbreak control were developed adequately; measures were taken promptly; and information was shared and disseminated smoothly.

On November 28, 2012, the eighteenth meeting on certification of polio eradication by WHO Western Pacific Regional Office (WPRO) was held in China. After comprehensive assessment of prevention and control of polio outbreak in China, the WHO WPRO certification committee confirmed that China set up a good model with characteristics of "timely response, prompt action, adequate measures and obvious effectiveness". It took only 3 months from report of the first polio case to the onset of last polio case in China.[1]

3.1 Background

Poliomyelitis (polio) is an ancient disease that human being has long been fighting against. There is a stele from BC 1580 to BC 1350, portraying a limp man with typical manifestation of the spinal cord sequelae of polio. In the early nineteenth century, there was a record of small scale polio outbreak in Europe, and in the late nineteenth century, polio outbreaks were reported in the United States. In the era when polio vaccine was unavailable, polio was the leading cause of lifelong disability in children, and was widely prevalent worldwide. There are 3 serotypes (I , II, III) of poliovirus, transmitted mainly through fecal-oral route. Only 1/100-1000 of poliovirus infections manifest paralysis, with the rest being asymptomatic infections, which is the major source of spreading the virus.

The goal of eradicating polio was adopted in 1988. The goal had been achieved in the World Health Organization (WHO) American Region, Western Pacific Region (WPR), and Europe Region in 1994, in 2000, in 2001 respectively. China is located in the WPR, with the last polio case detected in 1994. After 2000, when polio eradication was certificated in WPR, China had maintained a polio free status till 2010 by implementing the following strategies: 1) enhancing acute flaccid paralysis (AFP) surveillance of high quality; 2) improving and maintaining high routine immunization coverage of polio vaccine; 3) supplementary immunization activities (SIAs) with polio vaccines in priority areas; 4) timely and effective response to the outbreak.

As of 2010, there were 4 countries in the world where wild polio virus (WPV) was endemic, including India, Pakistan, Afghanistan, and Nigeria, among which India, Pakistan, Afghanistan share borders with China. There is no border for infectious diseases, therefore, no countries or regions are safe or protected as long as there is WPV in the world. It is not rare for WPV to spread or be imported from endemic countries to countries of polio free: according to WHO, WPV was imported to more than 40 countries during 2003-2010. In 2010, there were 1349 reported WPV cases in the world, of whom 232 were located in the endemic countries, and 1120 were reported by countries of polio free due to importation. Tajikistan, a neighboring country of China, reported 458 imported WPV cases and the WPV further spread to other three polio-free countries, namely, Russia (14 cases), Turkmenistan (3 cases) and Kazakhstan (1 case).

3.2 The shock

On August 25, 2011, the National Immunization Program (NIP) of Chinese Center for Disease Prevention and Control (China CDC) received a urgent report from the national polio laboratory that WPVs were detected from stool specimens of 4 AFP cases from southern Xinjiang.

No local WPV cases were detected for more than ten years in China since 1995. Did the lab results suggest that the polio virus had been quietly imported to China from abroad?

Experts from NIP developed corresponding preparedness plan for this emergency, focusing on the risk of importation and transmission of WPV in recent years. Xinjiang borders WPV endemic countries with frequent migration of population. Vaccination rate was relatively low in the southern Xinjiang where people in some areas had low immunity and there existed the risk of WPV importation. Paralysis cases due to WPV and local transmission might occur once the WPV was imported. At this critical moment, many questions needed to be answered, such as, when the virus was imported? How long had it been imported? How long would the spreading continue? What was the scope of the impact? How many cases were not yet found? How likely that the outbreak further spread out of southern Xinjiang?

China CDC sent the gene sequence data of the virus to WHO to determine where the WPV detected in AFP patients in the southern Xinjiang came from. China received a reply from the WHO 2 hours later that the virus was the same as WPV in Pakistan and the virus came from Pakistan, confirming that WPV was imported to China.

Box 3.1   General situation of Xinjiang

The Xinjiang Uygur Autonomous Region is located in Central Eurasia and northwest of China, with a total area of 1.66 million square kilometers, accounting for 1/6 of the total land area of China. Xinjiang borders with 8 countries, including Mongolia, Russia, Kazakhstan, Kyrgyzstan, Tajikistan, Afghanistan, Pakistan, and India, with a border line of more than 56 hundred km, accounting for 1/4 of the China land border line. Xinjiang is the largest province in China, with most bordering countries, and the longest land border line.

As of the end of 2014, there was a total population of 22 million in Xinjiang, of which ethnic minorities accounted for about 63%. There are 14 prefectures in Xinjiang, with the Tianshan Mountains dividing Xinjiang into northern and southern Xinjiang. There are 6 prefectures in southern Xinjiang, and 8 prefectures in southern Xinjiang. There are variations in geographical, ethnic and cultural characteristics between the northern and southern Xinjiang.

3.3   Emergency response

3.3.1   Notification

Notification of the outbreak is the required by the International Health Regulations (2005), and also a responsibility for all member countries. MoH sent the outbreak notifications to WHO, Shanghai Cooperation Organization, Association of Southeast Asian Nations (ASEAN), Japan, Republic of Korea, the United States, Pakistan and other neighboring countries or international organizations within 24 hours after confirming the occurrence of WPV importation in Xinjiang. Subsequently, the MoH regularly shared information with the WHO headquarter, WHO WPRO and WHO offices in the neighboring countries, the Global Polio Eradication Initiative (GPEI), Regional Certification Committee (RCC) on polio eradication, Technical Advisory Group (TAG), the National Certification Committees (NCCs) in other countries in WPRO and other organizations, with outbreak information disclosed openly.

3.3.2   Immediate actions

Outbreak trigged an emergency response. On the evening of August 25, the MoH immediately sent experts of epidemiology and public health to carry out the investigation of the outbreak in Xinjiang. At the same time, Health Department in Xinjiang established a leadership group. Results of investigation from the southern Xinjiang came continuously: more suspected polio patients were found through active search in hospitals of the southern Xinjiang, with not only pediatric patients but also adult cases being found. The situation is very urgent. It is critical to take adequate emergency measures as soon as possible to timely control the outbreak based on the situation analysis.

3.3.3   Reinforcements

The workload was heavy with tight time, so the MoH decided that the field work was conducted by governments at all levels in Xinjiang, with the experts from national level providing technical support.

The MoH organized the high-profile teams with management and technical expertise and sent them to Xinjiang to form joint working groups and expert groups together with local departments of Xinjiang Health Bureau. The first MoH team consisting of 71 epidemiologists, 18 clinical experts, 11 pathogenic experts from 14 provinces and cities went to Xinjiang on September 3. After a short training, the joint working groups, including MoH team, and Xinjiang's experts, immediately went to 5 prefectures, including Kashi, Hotan, Akesu, Bazhou, Kezhou, and provincial capital Urumqi to carry out the investigation. The working group worked round the clock to successfully complete the responsibilities on September 20.

Subsequently, 5 expert teams from provinces were sent to Xinjiang to assist in the investigation and handling of the outbreak. Under the leadership of local government and health administration department, experts cooperated closely with local teams to assist in community advocacy and mobilization, personnel training, AFP case searching, serum samples collection from healthy people, supervision and evaluation of polio vaccination SIAs. Satisfactory results were obtained. During the outbreak, ministerial level health officials visited Xinjiang for 9 times to lead and supervise the outbreak response work; China CDC sent a total of 100 professionals to guide and participate in response activities. The MoH mobilized a total of 500 person-times (each time about 15 days) of expert support to help Xinjiang. Experts contributed to the prevention and control of the outbreak by guiding and assisting the local team to carry out the outbreak responses and routine immunization.

3.3.4   Coordination & Cooperation

The MoH reported the outbreak to the State Council immediately after confirming the importation of WPV to Xinjiang. Vice Premier Li Keqiang gave instructions to stop the spreading of WPV as soon as possible. MoH initiated the second level emergency response, established a leading group with Health Minister as the head to lead the outbreak prevention and control efforts. At the same time a technical guidance group and a media communication group were set up.

MoH timely started the multi-sectoral coordination mechanism to inform the relevant departments of the outbreak information and to convene coordination meeting to discuss the response strategies. The senior working group, rapid response, close cooperation among the ministries, all played an important role in prompt and effective response to the outbreak. Every measure was quick, effective and orderly. A series of work went smoothly: MoH and MoE jointly issued a notice, requiring schools and kindergartens to monitor and report suspected cases of poliomyelitis; the State Administration of Quality Supervision Inspection and Quarantine timely issued a warning notification requiring to strengthen the port monitoring; the Ministry of Railways assisted in transportation of biosafety level three mobile laboratory from Beijing to Urumqi, to support the on-site emergent laboratory testing; MoH coordinated with China People's Liberation Army General Office, and the Civil Aviation Bureau to transport polio vaccines to Xinjiang; State Food and Drug Administration, CNBG ensured the vaccine supply for emergency vaccination; Institute of Medical and Biology, China Academy of Medical Sciences supplied monovalent polio vaccines for 2 rounds of emergency vaccination.

Xinjiang government established a leading group on polio outbreak on August 26, and multiple meetings were held to coordinate the prevention and control work. Xinjiang Government held three teleconferences on August 30, September 7 and November 12, with high-ranking officials such as Health Minister and the Chair of Xinjiang Government attended to provide the guidance on the outbreak response activities.

3.3.5　Investigation

According to the preliminary investigation and previous OPV immunization status, combined with comprehensive risk assessment, 2 kinds of outbreak control measures were taken based on the area type: the southern region, namely Kashi, Hotan, Bazhou Oblast, Akesu, and capital city Urumqi with large migrant population were selected as priority areas, and the rest prefectures were selected as general areas.

Case searching

A retrospective active searching of AFP cases was carried out in Xinjiang in order to find possible missed cases, and daily zero case reporting system was carried out to improve the sensitivity of surveillance. At the same time, quality of surveillance system was assessed, to evaluate the risk of missed reported cases. And a real-time AFP reporting system, which was the same with the reporting system of the notifiable infectious diseases, was implemented nationwide.

Initiation of daily Zero case reporting

Since August 28, 2011, Xinjiang began daily Zero case report system for AFP cases.

Any AFP case of any age found in all medical institutions in all 5 prefectures in southern Xinjiang and Urumqi were required to be reported daily, namely, all AFP cases should be reported, and the age group expanded from under 15 years old to all ages, the surveillance institutions expanded from the county hospitals to all hospitals at townships and above level, with a purpose to increase the sensitivity and timely detect all possible polio cases. In other areas of Xinjiang, all hospitals at county level and above should report all AFP cases under the age of 15 and suspected polio and atypical Guillain-Barr Syndrome (GBS) cases of any age.

Retrospective active search of AFP cases

In order to assess the severity of the outbreak, based on AFP routine surveillance, investigation and analysis were conducted to estimate possible underreported cases and to verify the reported cases. Therefore, a retrospective active search of AFP case was carried out in whole Xinjiang, as a supplementary approach to the routine passive reporting.

Active searching of AFP cases included active searching in hospitals, which was initiated on August 29, 2011, covering all AFP cases presented from January 1 2010 to August 28, 2011 in Xinjiang, and active searching house to house at the time of coverage survey and SIAs.

The scope of searching differed by prefecture: all hospitals and medical institutions at township and above level in 5 prefectures (Hotan, Kashi, Bazhou, Akesu, and Oblast) and Urumqi with large migrant population should be searched, covering all AFP cases at any age in 2011, and AFP cases below 15 years old and any suspected polio cases or atypical GBS cases at any age in 2010; the medical institutions above county level should be searched in 8 other prefectures, covering AFP cases under the age of 15, clinically suspected polio cases or atypical GBS at any age. During the searching in the hospitals, all outpatient and inpatient cases in Department of Neurology, Pediatrics, Internal medicine and Infectious disease were checked.

Virus surveillance

Nearly 99% of polio infections are asymptomatic, that is, the persons infected don't show clinical symptoms, but may discharge virus which may circulate and spread in the population and cause the outbreak. The virus may also survive in the environment for a long time and cause paralysis if infecting a susceptible person, leading to

clinical polio cases. Therefore, to monitor the carriage in healthy children and monitor the environment is a supplement to the AFP surveillance with the aim to improve
sensitivity of surveillance, timely detect the virus which may be circulating in the
population, and give clues about population infected.

Monitoring of virus discharged in healthy children

Stool samples were collected from healthy people in the 5 southern prefectures for virus
isolation before SIA. A total of 491 stool specimens were collected from August to October 2011, with 13 WPV infection detected by PCR. The infection rates by age were 4%
(4/101) among ages 1-4, 3.5% (8/226) among ages 5-14, 1.1% (1/93) among ages 15-39.
The distribution by prefecture was 2.5% (8/323) in Hotan, and 5.6% (5/89) in Kashi.

Environmental surveillance

China CDC transported a biosafety level 3 mobile laboratory to Urumqi on September 6, 2011, with adjustment of instrument and laboratory preparation completed
between September 7 and 11. On the evening of September 12, 25 water samples
collected from the 17 environment sampling sites (22 from Hotan and from Kashi)
were sent to the Xinjiang polio laboratory. On September 13, 17 environmental
samples were processed, and the eluent of environmental samples were obtained on
September 17. Virus isolation was performed on September 18 using SOAS WPVI
real-time fluorescence quantitative RT-PCR. The results showed that WPV1 were
detected in 2 samples in Hotan, and negative for the other 15 samples.

Vaccination assessment

Vaccination is the most economic and effective intervention to prevent polio, and is
also an important measure to stop the spread of the disease. Live attenuated poliomyelitis vaccine (OPV) is safe and effective, which has been used in China since 1960s
for routine immunization among children with a schedule of 2, 3, 4 months, and 4
years old. An annual 2 rounds of OPV SIAs were conducted in Xinjiang in children
under the age of 4 years. The scope of the outbreak could be estimated through the
vaccination rate survey, together with epidemiological data of the cases, which will
provide evidence for targeted age and geographical scope of the SIA.

Survey of OPV vaccination rate

From August 27 to September 1, 2011, a joint mission which consisted of national and

Xinjiang provincial experts conducted a rapid assessment of OPV coverage targeting children under 5 years old, with 2340 children investigated in Hotan city, Moyu, Hotan, Luopu, Yutian in Hotan prefecture. Less than 90% of children had vaccination certificates in the 5 counties, with only 72.2% in Luopu county, and less than 85% in Yutian and Hotan County. The coverage of routine OPV immunization was 93.2%, 90.3%, 86% for the 1st, 2nd, and 3rd dose of OPV respectively in 5 counties, with the lowest (78.8%) in Moyu, followed by Yutian and Luopu. The coverage rates of 2 rounds of OPV SIAs during March to April 2011 were 74.1%, 72.4% respectively.

At the beginning of September 2011, an extended rapid assessment of OPV vaccination rate in children aged 0-4 years old was conducted in 48 counties (city, district) in Akesu, Hotan, Kashi, Bazhou, Kezhou, Urumqi, and Yili before the emergency immunization. The coverage of the 1st, 2nd, and 3rd dose of OPV among the 6723 children was 97.13%, 95.75% and 93.65%. Among children above 4 years old, the coverage of the 4th dose OPV was only 46.43%, and only 15.93% in Hotan. The low coverage rate in some areas made it more difficult to rapidly block the spread of WPV.

Serum antibody surveillance

To understand the population immunity level, from August 27 to September 6, 2011, a total of 2611 serum samples from the general population were collected in the five southern Xinjiang prefectures before SIAs to test neutralizing antibody level against type I, II and III using micro neutralization assay. The results showed that antibody positive rate (antibody titer $\geq$ 1:4) were 90%, 90% and 82% for type I, II, III respectively. The positive rate for type I, II, III was 72%, 71% and 57% respectively among children under 1 year old (198), which was the lowest. The positive rate for type I, II, III was 92%, 93% and 91% respectively among ages 1-4 (435), and 97%, 97%, 90% respectively among those aged 5-14 (596), which was the highest of the subjects. The positive rate for type I, II, III was 88%, 90% and 79% among ages 15-19 (1059) and 94%, 90% and 83% among people over 40 years old (323).[1]

3.4 Actions

3.4.1 Containment

It is necessary to carry out OPV emergency immunization and SIAs as soon as possible in order to rapidly and effectively control the outbreak. In the response to the outbreak in Xinjiang, it is uncommon that the OPV emergency immunization targeted a wide range of age groups and a great number of people in the era of polio free. It was the first time for China to use monovalent OPV (mOPV) to conduct emergency immunization for the purpose of controlling an outbreak. Photos of emergency vaccination are shown in Figure 3.1-3.3.

Transportation of emergency vaccines(see Figure 3.1)

The southern Xinjiang is located in the northwest border of China, far away from central urban with climate changing fast. In order to ensure the vaccines being transported to the southern Xinjiang in a timely manner, MoH requested Chinese Air Force and civil aviation's support to the transportation of vaccines. A variety of transportations were used to ensure the timely deployment and arrival of vaccines in Xinjiang.

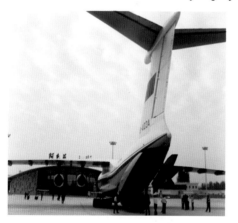
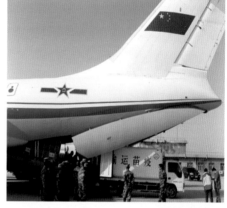

Air force transporting vaccines   Vaccines transported to southern Xinjiang

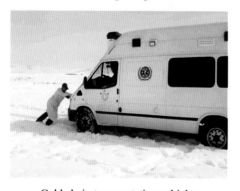
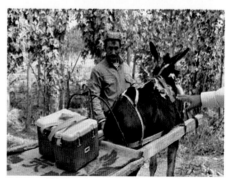

Cold chain transportation vehicles   Cart for vaccine transportation

Figure 3.1   Transportation of emergency vaccines

Extensive training and mobilization (see Figure 3.2)

Various forms of publicity were used to disseminate key messages of disease and the importance of vaccination, to alleviate social panic, improve the knowledge and increase awareness and compliance with vaccination.

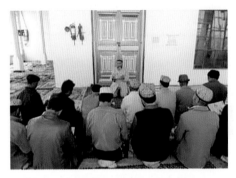

Religious leaders promoting prevention and control knowledge

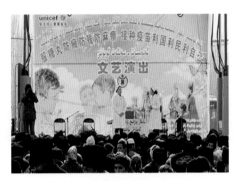

Vaccination programs

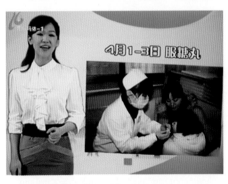

Television publicity on SIA

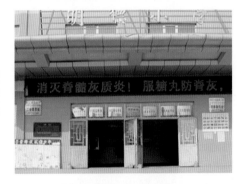

Vaccination campaign slogan

Figure 3.2 Extensive training and mobilization

Orderly organized vaccination site (see Figure 3.3)

Reasonable set-up of fixed point of vaccinations (POVs), combined with mobile POVs to provide different types of vaccination services for people in different areas. To ensure no missed vaccination (see Figure 3.4)

Children were marked after the vaccination, adults received written certificates after vaccination, every effort was tried to reach all people who should be vaccinated.

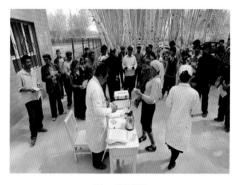

Fixed POV

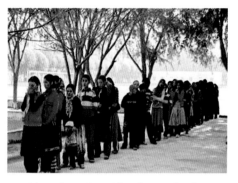

Line of people waiting for vaccination

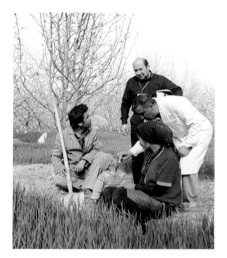

Mobile POV

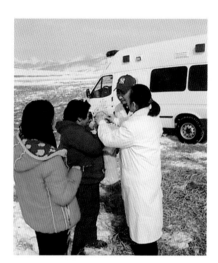

Mobile POV

Figure 3.3   Orderly organized vaccination site

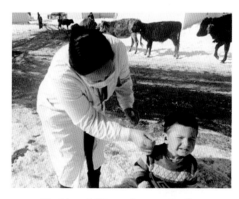

Marking children after vaccination

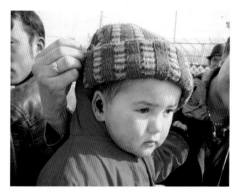

Children marked after vaccination

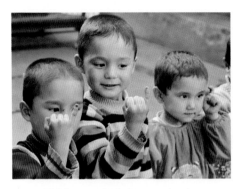

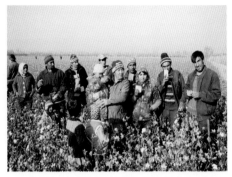

Children marked after vaccination   Cotton pickers with immunization certificates
in hand

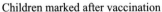

Figure 3.4   To ensure no missed vaccination

On August 29-31, 2011, a preliminary round of emergency tOPV SIA was conducted in primary boarding school, junior high school and kindergartens in Hotan where the cases were found and about 90,000 people were vaccinated.

In September and October 2011, the first two rounds of tOPV SIAs were conducted among children under 15 in 5 southern prefectures and Urumqi, also among children under 5 in other prefectures. The first and second round of SIAs provided vaccination for 3.9 million children, with a reported coverage of >99%. In September, the first round of SIA was conducted in southern Xinjiang covering adults aged 15-39, with a reported coverage of 99.4% and an estimated coverage of 95.7%.

In November 2011, the type I mOPV was used for the third round SIAs, covering the population under 40 years old in 5 prefectures in southern Xinjiang, under 15 years old in Urumqi, and under 5 years old in the northern region.

In March and April 2012, the fourth and fifth round of SIAs were conducted covering the population under 40 years old in 5 prefectures in southern Xinjiang, and under 15 years old in other areas. The fourth round SIAs used type I mOPV, while the fifth round SIAs used tOPV.

The cumulative OPV vaccines used for all five rounds of SIAs was 43.63 million doses (Table 3.1).

A rapid evaluation of vaccination rate was carried out after each round of SIA in order to evaluate the coverage of SIAs. The subjects being visited and evaluated was 11,155 for the first round, 3,601 for the second round, 9,071 for the third round,

23,414 for the fourth round, and 18,789 for the fifth round. The coverage rates were 99.4%, 99.6%, 98.1%, 91.8% and 98.5% for the 5 rounds of SIAs, respectively.

Table 3.1　Target population, time of emergency SIAs in Xinjiang from 2011 to 2012

Round	Target population	Time	Vaccinated people (×1000)	Vaccine type
First round Sep. 2011	Emergency vaccination Boarding school in Hotan	Aug.29-31	957	tOPV
	Children< 15 years old in southern Xinjiang and Urumqi Children< 5 years old in other prefectures	Sep.8-12		
	Adults (15- 39 years) in Hotan	Sep.13-17		
	Adults (15- 39 years) in other areas in southern Xinjiang	Sep.22-26		
Second round Oct. 2011	Children< 15 years old in southern Xinjiang and Urumqi Children< 5 years old in other prefectures	Oct.8-12	416	tOPV
Third round Nov. 2011	Adults<40 years old in southern Xinjiang Children< 15 years old in Urumqi Children< 5 years old in other prefectures	Nov.15-22	938	Type I mOPV
Fourth round Mar. 2012	Adults<40 years old in southern Xinjiang Children<15 years old in other prefectures	Mar.17-25	1023	Type I mOPV
Fifth Round Apr. 2012	Adults<40 years old in southern Xinjiang Children< 15 years old in other prefectures	Apr.16-25	1029	tOPV
In total			4363	

[§]Only five rounds of SIAs in children and four rounds of SIAs in adult included, emergency vaccination and supplementary vaccination for under-vaccinated not included in Hotan and Akesu.

3.4.2　Unified defense

MoH urgently requested all provinces to do a risk assessment so as to take appropriate measures to prevent the spreading of WPV from outbreak areas, and required Xinjiang to take immediate actions to block the spread of the virus.

After the wild polio outbreak was confirmed in Xinjiang, the rest of provinces in China also took measures to prevent WPV importation:

- Strengthen AFP surveillance.
- Polio vaccine immunization for under-vaccinated or SIA.
- Collect and test stools from healthy children.
- Strengthen the monitoring and vaccination among priority populations (such as cotton pickers) from WPV outbreak areas.

It was estimated that 2 rounds of SIAs were carried out in 23 provinces, 1 round of SIAs was carried out in 1 province. OPV immunization for under-vaccinated children was carried out in 6 provinces. The OPV vaccination in each province was significant for maintaining the antibody level of poliomyelitis in population and blocking the potential WPV importation.

3.4.3   Risk communication

China CDC established a communication and advocacy group on August 27 in response to the outbreak following the importation of WPV in Xinjiang, aiming to publicize knowledge on disease prevention and avoid public panic. The group was responsible for the surveillance and analysis of the needs by the general public, identification of key points for public communication, organization and development of health education materials, surveillance of public opinions and rumors, and tracking relevant information and giving feedback to the health authorities. Since August 28, call-in questions related to polio or Xinjiang outbreak from the public were collected daily through 12320 or other health hotline numbers. China CDC was responsible for the daily on-line network monitoring of news reports and posts at the main domestic and international media and communities and collecting concerns by the public and media. Experts were organized to prepare the answers to frequently asked questions on polio prevention and control, which was subsequently uploaded to the China CDC's main webpage on August 29 and September 23 to make sure all key messages were available to the general public.

China CDC experts also assisted the Xinjiang Health Bureau in developing a

public communication plan specific for this outbreak and instructed the local preparation of Uighur specific publicity and mobilization materials. Xinjiang Health
Bureau closely worked together with the Ethnic Committee to promote the health
communication activities in partnership with various departments whose tasks were
well defined. The TV script, pocket book on disease control and pilot work were
effective tools for disseminating core information to the public.

3.4.4   Norms

Based on international and domestic norms and experience gained from response
to outbreak, some technical programs and principles of response were carefully
developed by the national and local leading groups, to ensure that the outbreak
was promptly and orderly handled, and response activities were implemented
smoothly.

According to the emergency response level for WPV, national leading group
developed an emergency notice for surveillance of WPV importation, conducted a
survey of immune effect of polio vaccine, and made a risk assessment for transmission of the WPV. Xinjiang leading group developed 14 emergency programs to guide
prevention and control of polio outbreak, including program on active searching of
AFP cases, program of daily zero AFP case report, biosafety program for stool collection, transportation, and assay, program on transportation and distribution of vaccines for emergency immunization.

3.5   Truth

The whole picture of the outbreak was gradually coming to light along with implementation of the survey and response activities.

3.5.1   Time distribution of cases

21 cases of WPV cases had been reported with the first case occurred on July 3,
2011, and the last case occurred on October 9. There were two peaks of the outbreak,
the first showed up from July 3 to August 7, mainly in Hotan prefecture, and the
second took place from August 21 to September 9 in Kashi.

3.5.2   Space distribution of cases

21 cases were distributed in 4 prefectures in southern Xinjiang, with an overall incidence rate of 0.10/100,000 in Xinjiang and of 0.22/100,000 in four prefectures in southern Xinjiang. The incidence was the highest in Hotan (n = 13, 0.65/100,000), followed by Kashi (n = 6, 0.15/100,000), Bazhou (n = 1, 0.08/100,000) and Akesu (n = 1, 0.04/100,000).

3.5.3   Distribution of cases by demographic features

The incidence of WPV in male (0.29/100,000, n = 14 cases) was significantly higher than that of female (0.15/100,000, n=7). The incidence of WPV among children under 1 year old was the highest (3.46/100,000, n=6), followed by 1-4 years old (0.64/100 000, n= 4), 15-39 years old (n =10, 0.22/100,000), and ≥40 years old (0.04/100,000, n = 1). No cases were reported among 5-14 years old (Figure 3.5).

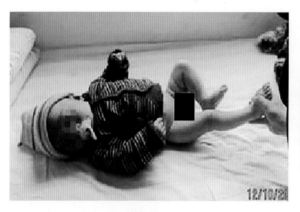 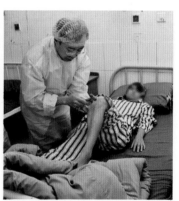

A pediatric case   An adult case

Figure 3.5   Among the 21 cases, 10 were under the age of 4 years, 11 were more than 15 years old. No cases were reported in the age group of 5-14 years.

3.6   Ending

The onset date of the first case was in July 2011, with a total of 21 cases of WPV reported. All cases were confined to 4 prefectures in southern Xinjiang. The highest incidence was reported in children less than 1 year old. Ten cases were under the age of 4 years, and 11 cases were over the age of 15 years, and no cases were aged 5-14 years. Of the 21 cases, 5 cases never received polio vaccines, 3 cases received 1 to 2 doses, and 5 cases received more than 3 doses, 8 cases with their immunization history unknown. After the outbreak, level II public health emergency response was initiated with a retrospective active searching and investigation of AFP cases, daily Zero AFP case reporting system was carried out, case definition and active surveillance in hospitals were expanded, rapid assessment of vaccination rate were conducted, and 5 rounds of polio vaccine SIAs were carried out.

Implementation of SIAs effectively brought the outbreak under control. The sensitive AFP surveillance found that the last laboratory confirmed polio case occurred on October 9, 2011. The sensitive AFP surveillance data indicated that no new cases were detected for the following 3 months after the last confirmed WPV case. The emergency response was terminated after comprehensive risk assessment, including environmental surveillance of poliovirus, antibody level survey in population. While maintaining the polio free status has to be continuously strengthened in order to prevent further importation of WPV. On April 10, 2012, WHO removed China from list of WPV endemic countries.

In order to assess the quality of the AFP case surveillance in China, the WHO expert group conducted an on-site evaluation of the Xinjiang AFP case surveillance system in June 2012 (Figure 3.6). Expert group concluded that AFP case surveillance system was sensitive in Xinjiang (incidence of non-polio AFP: 2/100 000), and

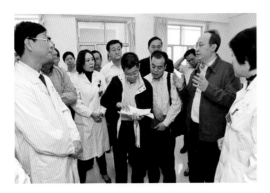
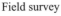

Field survey

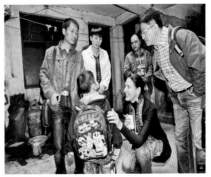

WHO in action

Figure 3.6 Expert group agreed after evaluation that the AFP surveillance in Xinjiang was sensitive with high quality, and concluded that: it was impossible for a circulating WPV not detected in Xinjiang.

well functioned, so that the system could timely detect potential or new imported WPV cases. No new WPV cases were found following the last case of paralysis on October 9, suggesting that the transmission of imported WPV had been blocked. According to the recommendations made by WHO expert group, AFP surveillance in Xinjiang returned from emergency status to routine one on August 1, 2012.

3.7 Praise

The rapid and effective emergency response to the outbreak due to the imported WPV successfully blocked the spread of the virus in a short time. On November 28-29, 2012, the 18th meeting of Certification Committee on Polio Eradication WPRO was held in Beijing (Figure 3.7). The committee concluded that China had successfully blocked the spread of imported WPV in Xinjiang, maintained polio free status, and created a China model for the investigation of and response to polio outbreak, and should be a model for other similar incidents. For example, preparatory work for SIA was completed within just 15 days, it only took one and a half months from confirming the first case (August 25) to the onset of last cases (October 9). Thanks to China's successful efforts, WHO WPR continued to be polio free.

WHO praised China model for outstanding decision-making and cooperation. During the outbreak, the MoH timely organized the expert groups and working teams and deployed them to the field to support Xinjiang's emergency response planning and implementation. MoH also provided guidance to neighboring provinces and other provinces for prevention measures based on the rapid risk assessment. Key measures like strengthening surveillance, improving geographic and population mapping for SIA, and using mOPV were all appropriate to confine the outbreak. The health departments and other governments departments at all levels provided strong support and cooperated extensively; China's collaboration with international organizations were enhanced; the responsibility for outbreak notification required by the International Health Regulations (2005) was perfectly fulfilled. This emergency response lasted for six months, which reached a new milestone in global polio eradication initiative (GPEI) strategic plan 2010-2012. The excellent investigations and responses well met the standards for WPV outbreak control established by the World Health Assembly in 2006.

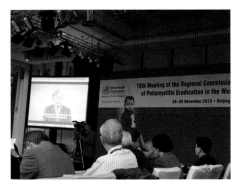

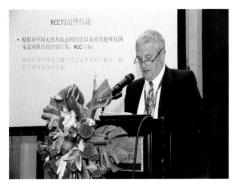

Dr. Shin Young-soo, Director of WHO WPRO gave a video speech at the opening ceremony: congratulations to Chinese government on outstanding achievements in the control of polio outbreak and prevent the spreading of WPV in the region.

Dr. Anthony Adams, Chairman of Polio Eradication Certification Committee WPRO, announced conclusions of RCC.

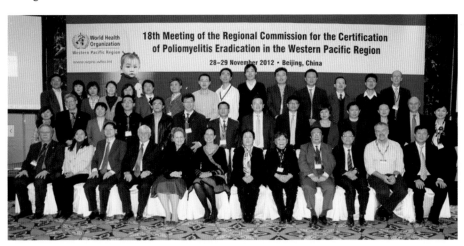

WHO WPRO staff and the Chinese team

Figure 3.7   On November 28-29, 2012, in the meeting of Regional Commission for the Certification of Polio Eradication in WPRO held in Beijing, it was announced that China was in a status of polio free, and the response to outbreak in China was praised.

3.8 Experience

The outbreak control set up a Chinese model in public health and enhanced the engagement of and cooperation among different ministries.

3.8.1   Technical basis for the outbreak response: an adequate emergency response plan

A good emergency response plan and its timely and effective implementation were essential technical basis for the successful control of the outbreak. On April 25, 2011, Chinese MoH issued *Emergency Preparedness Plan for Outbreak due to Imported WPV and VDPV (Trial Version)* in order to rapidly and efficiently respond to the outbreak caused by imported WPV and to minimize the threats caused by WPV related incidents. The disease prevention and control institutions conducted drills and exercises to practice emergency response actions for the possible importation of WPV. A hierarchical response principle is recommended in the plan, which describes the specific responsibilities of various departments during the outbreak. The MoH initiated a level II emergency response for the imported WPV outbreak according to the Plan and took actions to control the outbreak steadily and orderly, with each action supported by regulations.

Box 3.2   International Workshop on Polio Eradication

From July 21 to 22, 2011, China CDC and WHO co-sponsored an International Workshop on Polio Eradication, with Xinjiang CDC as the local host.

Participants included representatives from WHO headquarters and the European Region, Southeast Asia Region, Eastern Mediterranean Region and WPR, US CDC, US Agency for International Development and other international organizations, the key persons responsible for polio prevention and control from neighboring countries, including Pakistan, Kazakhstan, Russia, Tajikistan, Turkmenistan, Kyrgyzstan, Uzbekistan, India, Nepal, Burma, Mongolia, and Vietnam.

Participants discussed the challenges in global eradication of poliomyelitis; summarized the experiences and lessons learnt about the prevention of and response to importation of WPV; recommended to establish a platform for rapid exchange of information and data sharing via WHO; called on strengthening the cooperation among different countries or regions in data analysis, outbreak surveillance, quick release and notification of the outbreak information, especially for serious disease. WHO recommended to strengthen cooperation among countries through WHO or

---

other international organizations (such as the Shanghai Cooperation Organization) so as to jointly solve the problems encountered. Strategy of joint prevention and control among countries was advocated, so as to cooperate cross countries / regions once the outbreak of polio happens (including sending professional and technical personnel to provide support, communication network, resource sharing and providing emergency vaccines), and to promptly take emergency actions to block the spread of the disease.

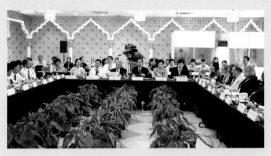

Figure 3.8   International Workshop on Polio Eradication was held on July 21-22, Xinjiang

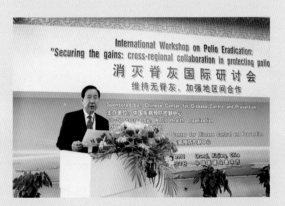

Figure 3.9   Wang Yu, Director General of China CDC, delivered opening speech.

3.8.2   Strong government leadership at all levels, clarification of responsibilities for all departments engaged in the outbreak responses

The MoH made a timely report to the State Council about the outbreak caused by imported WPV in Xinjiang. The MoF appropriated funds in time to support the response actions, with a total of 160 million Yuan allocated; The MoH and MoE jointly issued a notice requiring all schools and kindergartens to monitor and report suspected polio cases; Quality Inspection Bureau promptly issued a warning notice requiring strengthening the port surveillance; the Ministry of Railways assisted MoH with the transportation of biological safety level three laboratory from Beijing to Urumqi to carry out on-site emergency laboratory testing; the Chinese Air Force, the civil aviation and other departments transported vaccines to Xinjiang in time as requested by the MoH; SFDA, CNBG ensured the vaccine supply for emergent SIAs, Kunming Institute of biological products and China Academy of Medicine undertook the production and supply of type 1 monovalent polio vaccines for 2 rounds of SIAs.

3.8.3   The key to block the spread of WPV: take response actions quickly

After confirming the outbreak, the MoH and Xinjiang government took a series of prevention and control actions. In addition to the establishment of the leading group, notification of the diseases and investigation, other actions included: Deputy Health Minister in place in Xinjiang on August 27 to lead the overall outbreak response activities; OPV emergency vaccination conducted in schools of Hotan on August 29; publicity and social mobilization carried out on August 30; AFP surveillance and vaccination related training given on August 31; vaccines and refrigerated equipment for the first round of emergency SIA arrived in Xinjiang on September 2; Health Minister visited Xinjiang and joined the response on September 6 with a coordination teleconference held in Xinjiang; the first round of polio vaccine emergency SIA officially started on September 8. It took only 15 days from confirmation of the outbreak to the implementation of emergency SIA. Follow-up emergency responses or measures were also conducted effectively.

3.8.4   Timely detection of imported polio cases: high quality surveillance system

China established AFP surveillance system in 1991, with quality gradually strengthened and covering whole China with great efforts by CDCs and medical institutions

ment system (real-time online AFP surveillance system) based on the original AFP surveillance system. This system which was launched in 2012 was the world's first AFP case internet-based direct reporting system, with AFP case being reported in the same way as notifiable infectious diseases.

AFP surveillance information management system was a browser - server system, with module of case report, case information management and data analysis. Different authority is allocated to relevant persons for different modules. AFP surveillance information was entered through a personal computer's web browser via logging into the national server, with the authorization to specific persons to access the data, analyze the data and obtain the results on a real-time basis. China officially initiated AFP real-time reporting system on January 1, 2012. This system enjoys its advantages in timeliness, stabilization, safety and efficiency on epidemiological investigation of AFP cases in different regions, and was able to manage the cases in different regions.

3.10.2   Capacity of technical personnel at all levels improved

During the outbreak responses in Xinjiang, numerous training was conducted with capacity of technical personnel at all levels being improved. National experts conducted 21 trainings with 1,500 people participated and Xinjiang government conducted local trainings with 25,000 people trained. At the same time, cold chains, such as refrigerators and vaccine carriers were equipped for rural areas during the emergency SIA. POVs at village level were established, and a routine immunization service network was gradually established with the quality of routine immunization improved.

The last native WPV case in China was reported in 1994. Since then young public health personnel have not seen any polio cases and have little knowledge or experience about polio outbreak control. The experts of epidemiology, clinical medicine and etiology from other provinces were sent to Xinjiang to help with the case searching, zero case reporting, routine immunization and emergency SIA. By taking part in the response work, the experts also improved their knowledge of and practical experience about polio prevention and control. The capacity of disease control and prevention system was improved as a whole.

3.10.3   Immunization program in Xinjiang further improved

Local spreading of imported WPV in Xinjiang suggested that there were gaps in local polio vaccination and even the routine immunization program. After the outbreak, the MoH and Xinjiang made a thorough analysis of the local situation, and concluded that the main weaknesses included inadequate human resources on preventive vaccination in the rural; lack of sustainable mechanism to ensure the funding for CDC at grassroots level; and weak routine immunization. The vaccination was provided by home-visit in most areas of Xinjiang. The children in rural, remote areas and economy underdeveloped areas were not always covered effectively due to the large areas for limited service providers. The spreading of imported WPV in southern Xinjiang suggested that routine immunization was weak. Therefore, it is necessary to increase investment in immunization program, to stabilize the workforce and to improve the incomes of technical professionals. In the areas where the routine immunization is weak, the basis is to strengthen routine immunization. It is necessary to improve the network of routine immunization services, to establish a cold chain system with full coverage, to maintain the normal operation of the cold chain, and to implement the vaccination certificate checking system for school entry. After the outbreak, these problems have been addressed seriously by the government.

3.11 Summary

WPV was imported to China in 2011 and caused local outbreak in southern Xinjiang. There are two possible reasons for the spreading of the imported WPV. First, Xinjiang is adjacent to the WPV endemic countries (Afghanistan and Pakistan) with persistent risk of WPV importation; second, there existed population with low immunity, which was demonstrated by sero-epidemiology survey, vaccination rate survey and epidemiological study of WPV cases and clinical cases.

After the outbreak, Chinese MoH timely notified WHO and other international organizations, and received supports from WHO experts.

The outbreak was detected in time and response was made rapidly, mainly because the AFP surveillance system is of high quality; there is an emergency plan and technical plan for WPV importation; and the personnel are well trained for emergency response and drills were given.

The outbreak was quickly controlled with the following components recognized to be important: 1) unified leadership from senior administrative department of the government; 2) close cooperation among MoH and other Ministries; 3) international assistance; 4) timely and effective control measures; 5) effective SIA. It was appropriate to strengthen surveillance and to conduct emergency SIAs using monovalent OPV in Xinjiang covering the appropriate age groups. The health department and governments at all levels and other departments fully cooperated, with governments at all levels and relevant departments providing support and cooperation. China sent the notification about the outbreak to international organizations in a timely manner according to the International Health Regulations (2005).

After confirming the outbreak, the SIA preparation work was completed in just 15 days, and it took only one and a half months from confirmation of the outbreak (August 25, 2011) to the onset of last case (October 9, 2011), with the outbreak confined to the southern Xinjiang. The rapid and effective control of the outbreak brings up a China model, and WHO WPR continued to be polio free thanks to China's efforts.

References

1. Luo HM, Zhang Y, Wang XQ,et al, Identification and Control of a Poliomyelitis Outbreak in Xinjiang, China. The New England Journal of Medicine, 2013, 369(21):1981-1990.

2. http://www.wpro.who.int/immunization/news/china_1yr_polio_free/en/

3. Wang HB, Zhu SL, Zheng JS, et al. Sero-Survey of Polio Antibodies during Wild Poliovirus Outbreak in Southern Xinjiang Uygur Autonomous Region, China. PLOS ONE, 2014, 9(7):|: e80069.

Chapter 4

Remove Stigma of "Hepatitis B Country"

Fu-Qiang Cui, Guo-Min Zhang, Fu-Zhen Wang, Hui Zheng,
Ning Miao, Xiao-Jin Sun, and Ling-Qiao Zheng

February 24, 2014 is a day which is worth celebrating by Chinese public health society. On the day, Shin Young-soo, director of WHO Western Pacific Regional Office (WPRO), visited Beijing to give an award to Chinese government in recognition of China's remarkable achievements in the prevention and control of hepatitis B in children. Li Bin, Minister of National Health and Family Planning Commission (NHFPC), received the award on behalf of Chinese government. "Hepatitis B vaccination is the safest and most effective way to prevent hepatitis B virus (HBV) infection. Twenty years' experience in China has clearly demonstrated this practice." said Shin Young-soo, "Hepatitis B vaccination program in China significantly reduced the virus infection among children, which is one of the most important achievements in public health in China."

Prevention and control of hepatitis B in China was acknowledged by WHO experts as a great achievement in public health in the 21st century, which sets a global model. These achievements have been achieved within merely thirty years. What happened in these thirty years? As a " big hepatitis B country", what strategies were taken in China to effectively control the epidemic of hepatitis B? And what a tortuous road have these strategies gone through and finally been implemented? Zhao Kai, the former Director of Beijing Institute of Biological Products, a member of Chinese Academy of Engineering, and Wang Zhao, former Director General of Department of Disease Prevention and Control of Ministry of Health (MoH), led us to review the thirty years of war against hepatitis B in China.

In this chapter, we will share with readers about how hepatitis B was identified as a priority of public health, how hepatitis B vaccine was developed and advanced production lines was introduced, how hepatitis B vaccine was intergrated with hospital delivery and given to infants as the timely first birth dose, how the shortage of funds was addressed through international cooperation, how the safe injection was improved and blood born HBV infections was controled, etc. In the past 30 years, a great number of dedicated people have been working hard to achieve equity in hepatitis B vaccination and reduce HBsAg carriers in children with lots of touching stories.

4.1　Concern: Hepatitis B, a major and serious infectious disease in China

The human history is full of records of many diseases, including plague, smallpox, measles, influenza, etc., which took away countless lives. There is one disease which is not so notorious as the above diseases, but causes tremendous infections among humans and insidiously accompanies the carriers for many years, that is, viral hepatitis.

Viral hepatitis, especially hepatitis B, causes serious burden in China. During 1979-1980, Department of Disease Control and Prevention (CDC), MoH conducted a sero-epidemiological survey of viral hepatitis to understand the epidemic situation of hepatitis B in the Chinese population.[3]The survey covered 209 counties in 29 provinces, with a total of 138,000 people aged 0 to 80 years old being investigated. The survey showed that the prevalence of hepatitis B surface antigen (HBsAg) in the Chinese population was 8.75%. This was the first time the prevalence of HBsAg was estimated in Chinese general population. It was estimated that there were about 120 million people in China who carry the hepatitis B virus, equivalent to one hepatitis B virus carrier among ten persons. The hepatitis B carriers in China accounted for about 1/3 of the global total (350 million). According to the WHO's criteria, China was categorized as the high epidemic area (HBsAg prevalence rate ⩾ 8%) and natually was labelled as a " big hepatitis B country".

The national sero-epidemiological survey revealed the severe situation of hepatitis B in China, which aroused widespread social concern and drew attention of government officials. This survey also identified hepatitis B as a major infectious disease in China that needed to be prevented and controlled with strength. According to academician Zhao Kai: "The national Sero-epidemiological survey of viral hepatitis in 1979-1980 was led by Professor Liu Chongbai from the Institute of Viral Disease Control and Prevention. The serological markers were detected by reverse passive hemagglutination (RPHI) assay which showed that HBsAg positive rate was 8.83%. Later on, the reagent from Abbott Laboratories was used to confirm the results, which showed an adjusted HBsAg positive rate of 10.03%, a very high level. This result aroused the attention of the government and the healthcare field." After the survey, China initiated many scientific and technological research about hepatitis B from 1981 to 1995, which contributed to a better understanding of characteristics of hepatitis B and provided solid evidence for making specific control strategies.

4.2 Actively accelerate the research and development of hepatitis B vaccine

There is no cure for chronic infection of Hepatitis B virus. The chronic carriers usually carry the virus for life, causing heavy physical and mental burden on family and society. In the early 1970s, China initiated the development of plasma derived hepatitis B vaccine in extremely difficult conditions.

According to academician Zhao Kai, the research on plasma derived hepatitis B vaccine in China started in 1975. After 10 years of painstaking endeavors, the vaccine was finally approved in 1985. The conditions for research at that time were very hard. Hans Miller, a German medical expert and outstanding international doctor, and Tao Qimin, a professor at Beijing Medical University were the team leaders. The research team overcame the difficulties, conducted several hundreds of trials, and finally succeeded in developing the first batch of plasma derived hepatitis B vaccine on July 1st, therefore it was named "7571".[2] People's Daily reported this achievement as headline story in 1976.

For a country where hepatitis B was highly epidemic, the licensure of hepatitis B vaccine was a great scientific achievement, which could effectively block the spread of hepatitis B virus in the population and benefit Chinese people. The vaccine was a powerful weapon for the prevention and control of hepatitis B in China.

According to Zhao Kai, development of plasma derived hepatitis B vaccine received a total of three national awards and five Ministry level awards. It received the type A award of achievement in medical and health science from MoH in 1986, the 3rd award of national science and technology progress in 1987, the 1st award of national science and technology progress in 1988. Production technology and vaccination of plasma derived hepatitis B vaccine received the 1st award of science and technology progress from MoH in 1991. The development of expression system for genetic engineering hepatitis B vaccine won the 1st award of national science and technology progress in 1993, which is the highest reward in the field of science and technology in China. In 2008, South Weekend selected the top 10 Science and technology progress awards in China since the Reform and Open-up Policy 30 years ago, with hepatitis B vaccine ranking the 3rd. Hepatitis B vaccine was also the only selected achievement in medical science. In 1985, the plasma derived hepatitis B vaccine was launched under the advocacy of MoH, and it received the award of breakthroughs in science and technology field of "the 6th 5-year plan". Thereafter, the immune efficacy with large samples of hepatitis B vaccines in neonates was observed and evaluated from 1985 to 1990 in 5 provinces, namely, Hebei, Henan, Hunan, Shanghai, Guangxi with around 1 million people involved. At 9 years of follow-up after vaccination, the positive rate of anti-HBs antibody dropped from 73-93% in the first year to 45-48%, however, the average protection rate ranged from 83% (first year) to 92% (9 year), with almost no new HBsAg carriers detected in 5 to 14 years after vaccination, and anti-HBc antibody positive rate was also lower than 4%. These results fully demonstrated that the plasma derived hepatitis B vaccine induced reliable protection in neonates. However, considering the low production and high cost of plasma derived hepatitis B vaccine, and its safety indetermination with the risk of other blood-born infections, MoH stopped the production of plama derived hepatitis B vaccine in China on June 30, 1998, and its use ceased in 2000 (Figure 4.1).

Mass production of recombinant Chinese Hamster Ovary cells (CHO) hepatitis B vaccine was initiated in 1992, and officially launched in 1996[4]. The evaluation data of vaccine application showed that anti-HBs positive rate remained 71%-89% among the children at 2 - 6 years after being immunized with the recombinant CHO hepatitis B vaccine. Among neonates born to mother with both HBsAg and HBeAg positive, the protection rate in the first year after vaccination was 75%,with a more stable and better effectiveness of blocking vertical transmission than that when using plasma derived hepatitis B vaccine.

In 1989, production technology of recombinant yeast derived hepatitis B vaccine was introduced from Merck Co (Merck Sharp & Dohme) of the United States, with the vaccines produced by Beijing Institute of Biological Products under Chinese MoH and Shenzhen Kangtai Biotechnology Co., Ltd.. The domestically-made yeast recombinant hepatitis B vaccine was developed in China in 1995 and officially produced in 1996. According to a large scale survey, protection rate was 83% at year 4 after vaccination. Among newborns whose mothers were HBsAg and / or HBeAg positive, the protection rate was 86%, significantly higher than that with plasma derived hepatitis B vaccine.

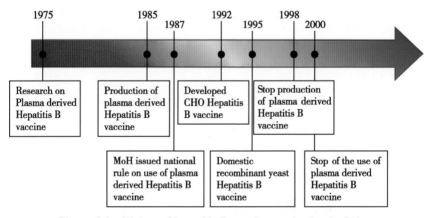

Figure 4.1   History of hepatitis B vaccine production in China.

Box 4.1   One promise, as good as gold[1] -- Merk company transferred the most advanced production technology of genetic engineering hepatitis B vaccine in the world to China 20 years ago

"In 1980s, hepatitis B is the most burdensome infectious disease in China, affecting 10% of people all over China, especially the farmers." Academician Zhao Kai recalled, "Facing this challenge, Chinese government was eager to find the best way to prevent hepatitis B and liver cancer".

In 1984, experts from China MoH visited Merck company in the US, and learnt the mature technology for yeast recombinant hepatitis B vaccine under development. "At that time, plasma derived hepatitis B vaccine was already in production in China, and China should introduce gene engineering technology if any new technology is to be introduced." academician Zhao Kai said, "through mutual visits and negotiations, in 1989 Merck and Chinese government reached a technology transfer agreement, Merck would provide the most advanced production technology of recombinant hepatitis B vaccine to China, and help China to establish the production facilities in Beijing and Shenzhen". In 1991, Chinese technicians visited Merck in the US for technical training. In 1993, China produced the first batch of recombinant hepatitis B vaccine using Merck technology.

Until now, these technologies and equipment were still operating efficiently and benefiting the Chinese people. Twenty seven years later in 2016, Roy Vagelos, former Merk CEO, a member of US National Academy of Sciences, the American Academy of Arts and Sciences, and academician Zhao Kai met again in Beijing, both of whom contributed to the technology transfer project (Figure 4.2). According to WHO, in 2016, 99% of Chinese children are protected from hepatitis B virus infection by vaccination.

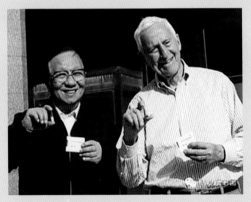

Figure 4.2　The 87 year-old Vageloos(right) and the 86 year-old Zhao Kai(left) held the latest batch of hepatitis B vaccine in hand, full of pride.

Box 4.2   The story about Miller and Chinese hepatitis B vaccine development[2]

Hans Miller was born in 1915 in a famous cultural city of Dusseldorf in German. He received Doctoral Degree in Medicine in 1939 in University of Basel, Switzerland, and then came to China to join the war against Japan. After the founding of New China, he changed nationality to China and joined the Chinese Communist Party to continue his contributions of wisdom and strength to the construction and people's health of New China, especially the research on hepatitis B and the development and use of hepatitis B vaccine. In 1989, he was awarded the Outstanding International Medical Worker by Chinese MoH.

Diagnosis and prevention of hepatitis B had been ranked high on the research priority list of Miller. He started to pay attention to this issue when he was in Yan'an. In 1973, under Miller's leadership, Professor Tao Qimin, with his laboratory team of Beijing People's Hospital which was affiliated to Beijing Medical College, successfully developed a sensitive blood cell with hepatitis B surface antigen, and established a sensitive detection method using assay reagent produced in China (Figure 4.3). However, Miller was not satisfied with the newly developed hepatitis B reagents. One day, he saw a message from an American magazine that the United States started hepatitis B vaccine research. Miller set up the goal for the research team, "we must develop hepatitis B vaccine in China, and we must make hepatitis B vaccination available in China".

The research conditions were very basic and poor at that time: a small aseptic room of only six square meters was separated from the warehouse, and equipment was inadequate, some 500cc bottles with glucose and iron shelf for venous transfusion. But everyone was full of vigor, courage and worked hard to overcome the barriers. After hundreds of trials, on July 1, 1975, the first batch of hepatitis B vaccine in China were produced.

Before putting into use, animal trial should be completed to ensure that the vaccine had no harm to the human and then clinical trials could be conducted. According to the literature, gorillas were susceptible to hepatitis B, however, there were no gorillas in China, and importation needs lots of foreign currency. Miller's research team didn't have this budget, and it seemed that this problem was unable to be solved. Research was interrupted once again. The newly developed hepatitis B vaccines could only be locked into the refrigerator.

When Miller learned that the current obstacle was that no animal experiments were able to be carried out, he talked to Tao Qimin, said: "please do the trial on me!" Dr. Tao was stunned, and rejected this suggestion flatly. Miller insisted: "I am over 60 years old, according to the Chinese culture, I am an old man already. I have been working in China for decades, all my things belong to Chinese people, I want to make some contributions to the Chinese people once more." Then, Miller further put forward the reason, he said earnestly: "I'm a doctor, a good candidate to experience the performance of the vaccine, please give me the vaccination!" Dr. Tao said firmly: "No." However, Miller's proposal inspired Dr. Tao. She secretly injected herself with the vaccine that night. When Miller knew this, he severely criticized Dr. Tao: "you are the leader of this discipline, if something bad happened to you, the impact on this project would be irreparable." Everyone observed and waited nervously, and the hard trail time passed. Antibody was induced successfully in Dr. Tao's body eventually. She survived. Inspired by Dr. Tao and Miller, the leaders of the hospital, the heads of the department, staff at the laboratory and the research group volunteered to receive the vaccine as the first group of subjects for the vaccine.

B.S. Blumberg, the Australian antigen discoverer and a US Nobel laureate, visited Tao Qimin's laboratory accompanied by Miller. He was surprised that the lab was so simple and crude! He couldn't imagine that, China successfully developed the vaccine on such a poor condition. Miller told him that the Chinese would continue to investigate the pathogenesis of hepatitis, cirrhosis, liver cancer and the relationships among them, and to identify measures and medicines to block the transmission and to make efforts to the eradication of hepatitis B eventually.

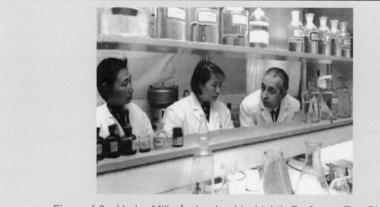

Figure 4.3   Under Miller's leadership (right), Professor Tao Qimin (middle), with his laboratory team were performing experiments.

4.3   In-depth investigation to evaluate the disease burden

At the same time when hepatitis B vaccine was developed, epidemiological special-ists carried out a lot of research, from risk factors of infection and disease burden to high risk population, to reveal the epidemiological characteristics of hepatitis B in China in the 1980s and 1990s, which provided valuable evidence for the develop-ment of scientific strategies for hepatitis B prevention and control.

During the period of "6th 5-year plan", and "7th 5-year plan", the research focused on the blocking of vertical transmission from mother to infant, which revealed that the earlier hepatitis B virus infection is the higher the risk of becoming chronic hepatitis is. For example, about 90% of perinatal infections will turn into chronic infections, and about 30% of infections in childhood (<6 years old) will turn into chronic infections, while only <5% of adult infections with no other underlying diseases will turn into chronic infections. In addition, according to the research and surveillance findings at that time, it was estimated that among 120 million hepatitis B virus carriers, 10% would result in liver diseases, such as chronic hepatitis, cirrho-sis and hepatocellular carcinoma. There were 12 million chronic hepatitis patients in China at that time and about 300,000 would die of liver disease each year, includ-ing about 160,000 liver cancer cases, majority of which were related to hepatitis B virus infection. The most serious problem was that at that time about 8% of pregnant women carried hepatitis B virus who might transmit the virus to newborns though vertical transmission, with about 0.8 - 1 million newborns being infected each year.

Thirteen years after the first national sero-epidemiological survey on hepatitis B, a second national sero-epidemiological survey on viral hepatitis was conducted from 1992 to 1995 in China,[5] with a similar result to the 1979 survey: 9.75% of Chinese people carried HBsAg, and prevalence rate of hepatitis B virus infection was 57.6%. Based on the result, it was estimated that there were 690 million Chinese people who had ever been infected with hepatitis B virus, of which 120 million were lifelong virus carriers. The survey confirmed once again that China was a highly endemic country of hepatitis B, and there were no improvements in hepatitis B infection situation over the past 10 years. No significant differences in HBsAg prevalence rate between the children aged 1-4 years old and the adults was observed, suggesting that most infection occurred in infants and the key strategy for prevention and control of hepatitis B in China was to vaccinate all newborns as early as possible.

4.4   Prevention first, making scientific decision

Although China was capable of producing hepatitis B vaccine, it was not until 2002 that hepatitis B vaccine was introduced into the national expanded Immunization Programme (EPI) and was provided free of charge for all neonates. This process was closely related to the Chinese economic development, and also reflected the remarkable consciousness of strategic decision from the health workers in previous generations.

In 1986, the plasma derived hepatitis B vaccine was produced and entered the market. MoH decided to launch the neonatal hepatitis B vaccination step by step. MoH issued *the National Interim Implementation and Management Guide for the Use of Plasma Derived Hepatitis B Vaccine* in September 1987 which standardized the use of hepatitis B vaccine, clarified that the protection of newborns was a priority, especially newborns delivered by HBsAg positive women, followed by children and other risk groups.

"Despite the guidance, at that time the hepatitis B vaccination was in an embarrassing situation." Director Wang Zhao said, "Because the general public lacked knowledge on hepatitis B vaccine, and hepatitis B vaccine was expensive, only 15% of the vaccines produced from 1986 to 1989 were used in newborns, while most of vaccines were used in cadre health care and staff in large enterprises as a welfare." In 1989, 24 members of the Chinese People's Political Consultative Conference(CPPCC), including Zhu Jiming, submitted a proposal to introduce hepatitis B vaccine into national immunization program gradually to the National CPPCC meeting, and wrote a letter to the Health Minister, Professor Chen Minzhang. In the proposal, 24 experts recommended to introduce neonatal hepatitis B vaccine into the national immunization program by regions step by step, and the first dose of hepatitis B vaccination for neonates should be provided in the Department of Obstetrics in hospitals to ensure vaccination within 24 hours after birth.

During the process of hepatitis B prevention and control strategy development, the former Minister of MOH, Chen Minzhang made undeniable contributions. Facing hundreds of millions of hepatitis B carriers in China, Chen Minzhang repeatedly mentioned in many meetings "As the Minister of MoH, it is my largest dereliction of duty and a shame if I ignore hepatitis B, and disregard the prevention of hepatitis B as a public health priority in a so-called big hepatitis B country."

Academician Zhao Kai recalled: "In 1985, hepatitis B vaccine was developed, and in 1987, the *National Interim Implementation and Management Guide for the Use of Plasma Derived Hepatitis B Vaccine* was issued. In order to implement this program, Minister Chen Minzhang held a hepatitis meeting in Dingfuzhuang in Beijing and established a leadership group for hepatitis prevention and control. From 1991 to 1995, Chen himself chaired five meetings on hepatitis B, to promote neonatal hepatitis B vaccination in China gradually."

Under Minister Chen Minzhang's support and encouragement, after rounds of expert consultation, in 1990 the MoH proposed that newborn hepatitis B vaccination strategy expand from urban to rural gradually. In the following 5 years, Minister Chen Minzhang chaired five specific meetings on hepatitis to promote the hepatitis B vaccination in Chinese neonates gradually: in the Xiangtan meeting in 1991, recommendations of national implementation of neonatal hepatitis B vaccination was proposed and the same year, the MoH issued *National Hepatitis B Vac-*

cine Immunization Implementation Scheme and *National Hepatitis B Vaccination Management Regulation(Interim version)*, in which it was determined that from January 1st 1992, hepatitis B vaccine would be introduced into management system of expanded programme on immunization (EPI) (Figure 4.4). The person who received the vaccine should pay for the vaccine and injection service fee with the importance of the timely first dose emphasized. The coverage data on timely vaccination of the first dose and full schedule was required to be collected and reported in accordance with the requirements of planned immunization. In Hangzhou meeting in 1992, the experiences of hepatitis B immunization were shared and the *National Hepatitis B Vaccine Immunization Program*" was further encouraged to be implemented. In Ji'nan meeting in 1993, it was proposed that hepatitis B vaccine immunization program expand from the urban to the rural. In TaiYuan meeting in 1994, it was clearly proposed that the strategic objectives for hepatitis B vaccination would be expanded from the urban to the rural. In Beijing meeting in 1995, the objectives of children EPI for 1996-2000 was put forward, the objective of coverage in neonates for hepatitis B vaccine in urban was more than 90% in urban areas and more than 60% in rural areas by 2000, and hepatitis B vaccination was included into EPI management system.

In the summer of 2000, Chinese Foundation of Hepatitis Prevention and Control, Chinese Academy of Medical Sciences and the Expert Advisory Committee of MoH co-hosted a meeting on strategy of hepatitis prevention. In total 50 well-known experts and scholars discussed about epidemiology of viral hepatitis and the strategic focus, objectives and measures for prevention of hepatitis B by vaccination in China. It was suggested that the vaccine be intergrated into the national immunization program (NIP). It was stressed that it was appropriate and urgent for including hepatitis B vaccine into NIP. At the same time, it was suggested that the central government allocate special funds to the 12 western provinces each year to purchase vaccines so as to ensure that the newborns would not miss the opportunity of vaccination due to poverty. 50 experts jointly drafted proposal for viral hepatitis prevention strategy in China, which was submitted to the offices of relevant leaders by He Luli, the Vice Chairman of National People's Congress (NPC), and aroused great attention by the Party and state leaders. After research and investigations by the relevant departments of the State Council, the Prime Minister Zhu Rongji, Deputy Prime Minister Li Lanqing gave instructions respectively, and in October 2001, MoH and Ministry of Finance (MoF) jointly issued a document *Notice on Introduction of Hepatitis B Vaccine Into National Immunization Program* (hereinafter refer to as the "Notice"). Governments at each province, autonomous region and municipality were responsible for the organization and implementation of the vaccination. Vaccine fee for eligible children would be covered by government at each province, autonomous region and municipality, with vaccination service fee paid by children's parents.

In August 2004, China revised the *Law of Infectious Disease Prevention and Control*, which clearly stated that a planned vaccination system was implemented with free NIP vaccination provided. In March 2005, the State Council issued the *Ordinance on the Management of Vaccine and Immunization*, which took effective on June 1st 2005. The Ordinance required that all NIP vaccinations should be free of charge to eligible children. So far, the hepatitis B vaccination for newborns in China was free completely. In addition, in order to strengthen the prevention of hepatitis B, hepatitis B was ranked as one of the four major infectious diseases in 2005 by MoH. And on January 28th 2006, MoH issued *National Plan for Prevention and Control of Hepatitis B: 2006 -2010.*

Based on the experience gained from neonatal hepatitis B vaccination, hepatitis B vaccination gradually expanded to other age groups in China. In 2009, the State Council identified six major public health service projects, with free hepatitis B catch-up vaccination for children under 15 years old who missed immunization

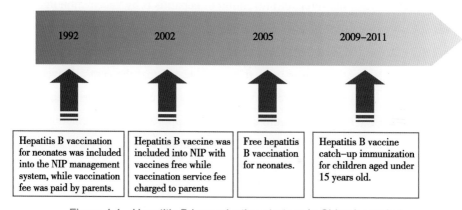

Figure 4.4   Hepatitis B immunization strategy in China by period.

as the first priority project, which required that within three years, children born between 1994 and 2001 who were not vaccinated with hepatitis B vaccines should be provided free hepatitis B vaccination service, to further reduce the hepatitis B infection rate and HBsAg carriage rate in this population.

4.5 To raise funds from various sources, to seek for international cooperation, and to promote the hepatitis B vaccination

Vaccines are divided into two categories in China: category 1 (traditional NIP vaccines) which are free of charge for children; and category 2, which are voluntarily vaccinated to children and charged to parents. Therefore, vaccination is partly influenced by economic conditions and parents' awareness.

Before introduction into NIP in 2002, hepatitis B vaccine belonged to category 2. The price of hepatitis B vaccine was relatively high, and vaccination service fee should be paid by parents, it resulted in a higher coverage of hepatitis B vaccine in the urban city and the rich eastern regions (90%) while a lower coverage in the poor western and middle regions (<40%).

4.5.1 Establishment of financing mechanism with multiple sources, solving the shortage of funds[6]

Minister Chen Minzhang was the founder of Chinese Foundation of Hepatitis Prevention and Control (CFHPC). The establishment of the foundation was the crystallization of Minister Chen's painstaking efforts.

In 1990s, the promotion of hepatitis B vaccination was difficult in rural, remote and poverty-stricken areas in China. At that time single dose was cost more than ten Yuan, and it took nearly thirty to forty Yuan or up to fifty to sixty Yuan in some instances for the full schedule. This was a big expenditure in rural and remote poverty-stricken areas. At that time, due to the inadequate economic development, the government was unable to pay all the costs of neonatal hepatitis B vaccination, Minister Chen thought of the creation of a foundation for hepatitis prevention and control in China, which would raise funds from domestic and abroad, to promote the hepatitis

B vaccination in rural, remote and poverty-affected areas in China. Therefore, Chen decided to establish CFHPC, which focused on promotion of hepatitis B vaccination in rural, remote and poverty-stricken areas in China.

In November 1995, the MoH formally submitted the application to the central bank to establish the CFHPC, and received the approval by central bank in June 1996. On August 22nd 1998, with the support of Premier Zhu Rongji, Vice Premier Li Lanqing and other national leaders, CFHPC was successfully registered in China. On November 24th 1998, CFHPC was formally inaugurated.

A few months after CFHPC was founded, Minister Chen Minzhang died of illness. Out of great concern to the national health and respect to Minister Chen, He Luli, Vice Chairman of National People's Congress, served as the Director General of the CFHPC. Very soon, the CFHPC received lots of donation and vaccines from a number of domestic and foreign associations and enterprises. In 2000-2002, CFHPC raised millions of dollars to provide free hepatitis B vaccines for 600,000 newborns in 35 remote poverty-affected counties through the poverty alleviation project, which increased the hepatitis B vaccination rate in these counties from 30% to 95%. In 2002 more than 50 experts jointly recommended to implement hepatitis B vaccine program, promoting the introduction of free vaccination policy. In 2005, the CFHPC investigated 2109 hepatitis patients in 28 hospitals and drafted the report of hepatitis and the related problems in China, which made in-depth analysis on the epidemiology, treatment, immunity protection, public awareness, social attitude and policy environment of hepatitis. Specific measures and recommendations were put forward and were fully recognized by the senior leadership. In 2007, CFHPC organized social campaigns and provided special funds to investigate on hepatitis B prevention and control among 729,000 college students in 60 universities of 14 provinces (cities, districts), providing important basic information for the establishment of national standard.

Box 4.3 The story of Chen Minzhang, final proposal in the bed in hospital

Professor Chen, a student of famous current Chinese medical scholar Zhang Xiao-qian, was the former Dean of Union Hospital. He stepped out of the hospital and took charge of public health in the Health Ministry.

In March 1998, Zhu Rongji visited Minister Chen in Union Hospital who just finished surgery due to pancreatic cancer. After surgery, Chen was weak with no strength for speech, and with a layer of fine sweat oozing from time to time in his pale face. Despite this, he still said his last wish and request with pains to former Premier Zhu who bent to listen: please approve the establishment of CFHPC so as to cooperate with the government to control hepatitis by providing all the children, especially those in remote and poor areas, whose parents couldn't afford, with timely hepatitis B vaccination. He sincerely stressed to Zhu that this was an urgent matter for China, and also his last request.

On November 24th 1998, a day with beautiful weather, CFHPC was formally established in the Great Hall of the People! This was the day Minister Chen waited for days and nights and was the crystallization of his painstaking efforts. However, as the founder of CFHPC, Chen had no strength to go out of the bed due to illness. He asked his secretary to donate all the income received for book writing, a total of 30,000 Yuan, to CFHPC on his behalf, the first personal donation received by CFHPC, and the largest individual donation so far received by CFHPC. White clouds witnessed his warm heart.

4.5.2 Strengthening international cooperation, obtaining financial and technical support

In 2002, with the help of experts from WHO, PATH, US CDC and other international organizations, CHFPC, Chinese government and GAVI determined to provide free hepatitis B vaccines for children in poor counties in middle and western China, and to implement safe injection. China GAVI project provided a funding of 76 million US dollars, with 50% provided by MoH/GAVI project, and 50% provided by the Chinese government.

The GAVI project covered the costs of all hepatitis B vaccine and syringes in 22 counties during 2002-2007, as well as part of the cost of Auto Disable (AD) syringes for other NIP vaccines. During the implementation of GAVI project, some other activities were also ongoing, including research on strategy for increasing the coverage of first dose of hepatitis B, social mobilization and advocacy, training, hepatitis B serological epidemiological survey, supplementary immunization for children missing vaccination opportunities. In 2010, the final assessment of GAVI project showed that hepatitis B vaccination rates achieved the target of 85% in 98% of project counties; timely vaccination rate for the first dose of hepatitis B vaccine achieved the target of 75% in 80% of project counties, and AD syringe was introduced in all the GAVI project counties. GAVI Global Representative Mark Kane said that the effective management of the GAVI project in China, such as the establishment of the project office and project executive advisory group which are responsible for supervision, sets a good example for other countries for implementing global GAVI project. Former Health Minister Chen Zhu also highly praised the GAVI project in China: the great success of GAVI project in China contributed to the control of hepatitis B in China; provided useful references for other infectious diseases, and explored a model for international cooperation, which is one of the most successful models in the field of global public health in the 21st Century[7].

4.5.3 Continue to increase government funding, to ensure sustainable development

From 2002 to 2005, the central government provided 36 million Yuan annually to support GAVI project provinces.[7] The 22 project areas provided a counterpart funds with a total of 180 million Yuan from 2002 to 2006, accounting for about 30% of the syringe funds and about 100 million Yuan as the performance budget. In 2004, central government provided a total of 112 million Yuan as vaccination allowances, 1 Yuan per dose, for Midwest regions through transfer payments. In 2005, this vaccination subsidy per dose increased from 1 Yuan to 2 Yuan in the national poverty alleviation counties, minority ethnic counties, and border counties. In 2005, the hepatitis B specific program provided 12 million Yuan to support vaccination for those missing opportunities and training, and in 2006, 15.4 million Yuan were allocated to support vaccination for those missing opportunities and surveillance. In 2007, the NIP vaccine list expanded, and the central government provided free hepatitis B vaccination for all newborns in China.

4.6 To improve the high hepatitis B vaccine coverage in China

4.6.1 Implementation of routine immunization

In order to carry out routine immunization of hepatitis B vaccine, and to ensure timely vaccination of the first dose, China health administrative departments clearly put forward the principle of "the person who delivers newborn should be responsible for the first dose of hepatitis B vaccine" (Figure 4.5) and a "three-copy letter" system was used for hepatitis B vaccination.

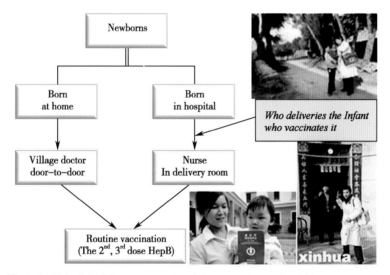

Fig 4.5   Principle "the person who deliver newborn should be responsible for the first dose of hepatitis B vaccine" in China

In 2002 when the hepatitis B vaccine was intergrated into children's immunization program, delivery in hospital was relatively low in China especially in the western regions and some minority groups in remote areas where a high proportion of newborns are delivered at home. Given this situation, close cooperation and information exchange between maternal and child institutions and points of vaccination (POVs) was enhanced. A routine monthly meeting mechanism was implemented with the person responsible for delivery in medical institutions, staff in POVs or village doctors attending. During the meetings medical institutions will exchange with the staff in POVs or village doctors of the pregnant information, including name, address, expected date and place of delivery, etc., so as that the staff in POVs or village doctors will learn the pregnant women who may give birth at home, and then go to the family in advance to communicate and learn the newborn's information, to improve timely vaccination rate of hepatitis B vaccine in children born at home (Figure 4.6). All rural doctors should be given appropriate incentives for timely vaccination of newborns born at home.

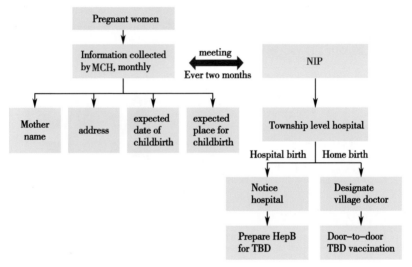

Figure 4.6   Close cooperation between immunization departments and maternal and child departments to improve the timely vaccination of first dose hepatitis B vaccine.

The full schedule of hepatitis B vaccine include 3 doses, with the first dose provided mainly by obstetrics and gynecology department in hospital, or by midwives or POV at village or community for newborns delivered out of hospitals; with second and third dose by POV at village or community where the newborn lives. How to achieve a seamless connection between the first dose and the remaining doses is a practical problem encountered. A "3-copy letter for hepatitis B vaccination" was used, namely, the information of first dose is transferred to POV through "3-copy letter for hepatitis B vaccination" for reference of the second dose. The "3-copy letter for hepatitis B vaccination" was filled after the first dose of hepatitis B vaccine by the hospital, with one copy kept by the hospital, one copy taken by newborn's guardian to be transferred to POV at village or community; and one copy kept in local county CDC. The "3-copy letter for hepatitis B vaccination" includes newborn's name, parents' name, address, date of birth, delivery hospital, the date of first dose of hepatitis B vaccine. POVs will provide vaccination card, certificate and fill in records according to the "letter". The local county CDC will check the vaccine number according to the "letter". The "letter" system contributed to the orderly connection and management of hepatitis B vaccination.

4.6.2 Combine hospital delivery with first dose of neonatal hepatitis B vaccine

Timely vaccination of the first dose of hepatitis B vaccine and completion of the schedule is critical to ensure the success of hepatitis B vaccination. The most valuable experience in promoting timely vaccination of the first dose hepatitis B vaccine in China is to strengthen cooperation between maternal and child health institution and NIP, to ensure timely vaccination of the first dose hepatitis B vaccine through increasing the rate of hospital delivery.

In 1980s, the delivery rate in hospital in China was very low, with the vast majority of pregnant women giving birth at home. According to data in 1985, average delivery rate in hospital was only 43.7% in China.[8] From January 2000, the MoH, the State Council Working Committee on Women and Children, MoF conducted a project on reduction of maternal mortality and elimination of neonatal tetanus in the Midwest rural China (referred to as "Jiangxiao Project"). The project included all areas of low economic development in the Midwest China, covering a population of about 400 million. By the end of 2005, the total funds for poverty relief project was 160 million Yuan, including 72.89 million from central government. A total of 730,000 pregnant women below poverty line were funded for hospital delivery, for treatment of obstetric complications and safe delivery service, an average of 200 Yuan for each delivery in hospital. In 2009 when medical and health system reform was further deepened, Chinese government issued the *Guideline on further improving of delivery in hospital in rural areas*, and other important documents, including providing maternal and child health services, such as delivery in hospital, as well as providing reimbursement of 500 Yuan per delivery in hospital by the new rural cooperative medical scheme (NCMS) project. As of 2011, 7.9 billion Yuan was invested to support the hospital delivery in rural areas, with about 22.6 million women benefiting from it.[9] As of 2013, China's NCMS project covered 97% of areas in China.

Implementation of the "Jiangxiao project" and the NCMS project, successfully increased the hospital delivery rate from 78% in 2002 to 99.7% in 2014,[8] effectively reducing the maternal mortality and the incidence of neonatal tetanus, and increasing the timely vaccination rate of the first dose hepatitis B vaccine in middle and western China significantly (Figure 4.7).

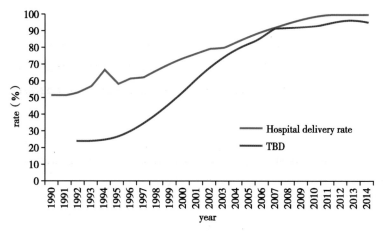

Figure 4.7　Hospital delivery rate and timely vaccination rate of first dose hepatitis B vaccine (TBD) in newborns in China, 1990-2014

4.6.3　System of checking immunization certificate before entering school provides the second opportunity for hepatitis B vaccination

According to the *Law on Infectious Disease Prevention* and the *Vaccine Distribution and Vaccination Regulations* issued by State Council, immunization certificate system for children is implemented in China, requiring all children be vaccinated in accordance with the NIP schedule.

In order to reduce the risk of infectious diseases in schools, health departments and education departments closely cooperated to develop relevant policies requiring that the immunization certificate be a requisite for entering kindergartens and schools. Checking immunization certificate is included into the standard procedure for entering kindergartens and schools. Those with no immunization certificates or failing to receive all doses of NIP vaccines should go to POVs to supplement the certificate and complete the missed vaccine(s).

4.6.4 Extensive social mobilization and health education to improve the level of public knowledge

In order to facilitate the inclusion of hepatitis B vaccine into NIP, to improve people's understanding about serious threats of hepatitis, and to enhance the hepatitis prevention and treatment measures, the MoH determined that the theme of the National Immunization Day of April 25th must be related to hepatitis B vaccination since 2002. All mass media such as radio and television, newspapers, magazines, posters were used to disseminate key messages about hepatitis B vaccination and prevention, with the aim to improve the awareness and knowledge of health staff and parents/guardians. In 2011, the WHO designated July 28th as the World Hepatitis Day, and Chinese government responded actively through utilization of the World Hepatitis Day to carry out social mobilization for prevention of hepatitis B, and to improve the basic knowledge on hepatitis so that parents actively participate in the initiative of vaccination.

4.6.5 Implementation of comprehensive prevention and control measure to reduce the spread of hepatitis B virus by blood

With the implementation of *Law on Infectious Disease Prevention and Control, Law on Blood Donation, Regulation on Management of Medical Institutions*, the following measures were taken to prevent the transmission of hepatitis B via blood: 1) Strengthening the supervision and management of institutions for blood collection and blood products; 2) Promoting the use of disposable syringes in medical treatment and prevention, and promoting AD syringes when appropriate, with repeated use of disposable syringes prohibited; 3) Strengthening the management of medical equipment; 4) Strictly implementation of the working standards and technical rules for prevention of iatrogenic transmission; 5) Strengthening the comprehensive measures of prevention and control of blood borne diseases during treatment.

4.7   Thirty years of efforts resulting in remarkable achievements

4.7.1   Vaccination rate of hepatitis B vaccine increased significantly

The average coverage of the timely first dose of neonatal hepatitis B vaccine increased from 39% in 1992 to 94.96% in 2014, and coverage of full doses of hepatitis B vaccine increased from about 30% in 1992 to 99.39% in 2014 (Figure 4.8) through comprehensive prevention and control strategies focusing on hepatitis B vaccination in the past 20 years since 1992. In 2010, the final assessment of MoH / GAVI project showed that the coverage of full course of hepatitis B vaccine rose from 71% in children born in 2002 to 93% in children born in 2009, the coverage of the first dose of hepatitis B vaccine rose from 60% in children born in 2002 to 91% in children born in 2009.

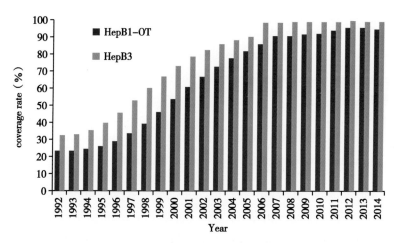

Figure 4.8   Hepatitis B vaccination coverage (source from 2006 and 2014: national hepatitis B serological survey).

The newborns are the priority for prevention of HBV infection. Besides newborns, those children with no immunity are still susceptible to HBV, who will be effectively protected from infection by providing supplementary immunization. Therefore, a systematic, step-by-step hepatitis B immunization program was carried out for children in addition to newborns on the basis of neonatal immunization since

2005. From 2002 to 2006, supplementary immunization for those missing vaccination was carried out in 16 provinces, autonomous regions and municipalities with 8.2 million doses used for children born in 2002-2005. Supplementary Hepatitis B vaccination was conducted in Qinghai, Jiangsu, Zhejiang, Tianjin, Shandong in 2007, covering children under 15 years old, with 300,000 people vaccinated in Qinghai; 1.3million doses used in Jiangsu (2 rounds); 1.51 million doses used in Zhejiang; 1.3 million doses used in Tianjin; and 3.83 million doses used in Shandong. In addition, MoH provided supplementary hepatitis B vaccination in 2009-2011 for children born in 1994-2001 who didn't complete the full schedule to promote the equity of basic public health services, and to accelerate the control of hepatitis B. During the three years of the project, 68.31 million people who were born from 1994 to 2001 were provided supplementary vaccination. It can be assumed that by the end of 2011, all children born after 1994 in China were provided with free and full hepatitis B vaccination.

4.7.2　HBsAg prevalence rate decreased significantly

Hepatitis B immunization strategy promoted the prevention and control of hepatitis B in China greatly, with the coverage of hepatitis B vaccination greatly increased, and hepatitis B HBsAg prevalence rate decreased significantly among young age children. In 2006, the third national serological epidemiology survey on hepatitis B was conducted which showed that HBsAg carrier rate was 7.18% in China, decreased by 26.36% compared with that in 1992. HBsAg carrier rate in children aged 1-4 years old was 0.96%, decreased by 90% compared to that in 1992 (9.67%).[10] Through the neonatal hepatitis B vaccination, 19 million HBsAg carriers were prevented since 1992 in China, and 80 million infections in children were avoided.

Based on results from the national hepatitis B serological epidemiology survey conducted in 2006, MoH submitted an application to WHO Western and Pacific Regional Office in 2012 for the verification of achieving objectives of hepatitis B control. The expert panel reviewed the publications and documents submitted by China. Expert group reached a unanimous conclusion after review: HBsAg carriage rate (survey in 2006) has dropped to <1% among children born after 1999. Therefore, China has successfully achieved the objective to reduce HBsAg carriage rate among children under 5 years old to less than 2% by 2012 proposed by WHO. On

March 6th 2014, the current Minister of NHFPC, Li Bin said in NPC and CPPCC: "HBs Ag positive rate in children under 5 years old was reduced from previous 10% to current less than 1%. We have now removed the 'hat of big hepatitis B country'".

After the recognition by WHO, a fourth national hepatitis B serological survey was conducted in November 2014 in China, with people aged 1–29 years being investigated, i.e. those people born after the vaccine approved in China in 1986. The findings are even more exciting: the prevalence of HBsAg among people aged 1–29 in China was 2.6%, the prevalence of HBsAg was 0.3%, 0.9% and 4.4% respectively among people aged 1–4, 5–14 and 15–19 years old. The prevalence of HBsAg among children aged 1–4 years old decreased by 97% and 67% compared with 1992 and 2006 respectively. The prevalence of HBsAg in children aged from 5–14 years old decreased by 91% and 61% respectively compared with those in 1992 and 2006(Figure 4.9).

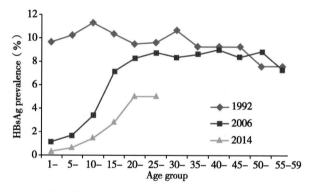

Figure 4.9   Significant reduction of HBsAg in young children from 1992 to 2014: 3 national Hepatitis B serological survey in China.

4.7.3   Hepatitis B vaccination results in enormous economic benefits

The treatment of Hepatitis B is expensive and complicated, which drove many families into poverty in China. Annual direct medical cost for treatment of hepatitis B and related liver diseases amounts up to tens of millions of Yuan. Neonatal hepatitis B vaccination effectively blocked the perinatal transmission of HBV, so as to avoid economic loss due to HBV infection and chronic liver disease, cirrhosis and liver cancer and other serious diseases. At the same time, vaccination greatly reduced hepatitis B carriers rate in the population, which brought along an enormous economic benefits and social benefits at population level. According to the health economics models,[11] a total of 65.3 million people were protected from HBV infection through hepatitis B immunization strategy in children during 14 years from 1992 to 2005, including 13 million acute infections and 650,000 chronic infections, 60,000 liver cirrhosis and 6,000 liver cancer cases. In China, around 5.348 billion Chinese Yuan were provided for Hepatitis B vaccination from 1992 to 2005, the total benefits gained were 272.825 billion Yuan, with net benefit as 267.477 billion Yuan. The cost for each infection averted was 81.99 Yuan while the benefit of one Yuan being invested created 51.01 Yuan in return.

References

1. https://www.ishuo.cn/doc/ybnoiqqf.html.

2. Shen Haiping. Miller and development of hepatitis B vaccine in China. Archive Spring/Autumn, 2015; 12: 12-6.

3. Li Yu. Epidemiology of viral hepatitis in China. Chin J Microbiology and immunology,1986; sup: 1-14.

4. Liang Zhenglun. Research and development of hepatitis B vaccine in China. Chin J Microbiology and immunology, 2013; 33(1): 11-4.

5. Dai ZC, Qi GM, editors. Virual Hepatitis in China(Part One): Seroepidemiological Survey in Chinese Population , 1992-1995. Beijing: Scientific and Technical Documentation Press, 1997.

6. http://www.people.com.cn/GB/paper503/5575/571315.html.

7. Kane MA, Hadler SC, Lee L, et al. The inception, achievements, and implications of the China GAVI Alliance Projecton Hepatitis B Immunization. Vaccine, 2013; 31(supplement 9): 15-20.

8. National Health and Family Planning Committee. Annuals of Health and Family Planning in China. 2015.

9. Yang Zhiyong, Wang Zaoli. Policy of Subsidy for Delivery in Hospitals for Maternal in Rural China and Cross-sectional Analysis. Chi. J of Health Economics, 2013; 32(3): 64-7.

10. Ministry of Health,Chinese Center for Dsease Control and Prevention. The National Report of Hepatitis B Sero-survey in China. Beijing: People's Medical Publishing House, 2010.

11. Zhang Shunxiang, Dang Rubo, Zhang Weidong, et al. Effectiveness of Hepatitis B Vaccine and Health Economics/Policy Analysis ofCurrent Strategy. Chin. J of Epidemiology,2008; 29(10): 1003-8.

Chapter 5

An outbreak of human Streptococcus suis serotype 2 infections presenting with toxic shock syndrome in Sichuan Province

Wen-Wu Yin, Li-Ping Wang, Zhong-Jie Li, Hong-Jie Yu, and Wei-Zhong Yang

5.1 Investigation of a strange disease

Between July 11 and 12, 2005, the third hospital in Ziyang Prefecture of Sichuan Province reported 2 suspected cases of hemorrhagic fever with renal syndrome to Yanjiang District Center for Disease Prevention and Control (CDC), Ziyang Prefecture, with no epidemiological evidence. The District CDC conducted a retrospective survey in the hospital and found that the hospital admitted and treated 4 similar cases in the past half month, among whom 2 died, 1 lost to follow up with outcome unknown (spontaneous leaving hospital), 1 was still on treatment. Three patients were located in Yangjiang district, and the other 1 came from the neighboring county. All patients had a history of contact with or eating meats of pigs or sheep that had died of unknown reasons. The cases are distributed widely in geography, with no contacts among each other. The clinical manifestations included sudden high fever, malaise, nausea, vomiting, followed by hypotension, syncope, shock, as well as petechiae in face, upper arm, and chest (Figure 5.1). Clinical investigations showed a progressive increase of white blood cells, progressive decrease of platelets, and increase of urine protein.

On July 13, 2005 Ziyang CDC staff went to the hospital to investigate and collect blood samples which were then sent to the Sichuan Provincial CDC for

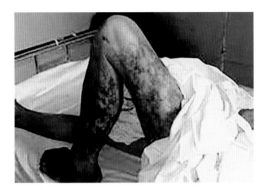

Figure 5.1   A Streptococcus suis patient with toxic shock syndrome with severe bleeding in the skin and disseminated intravascular coagulation.

testing. Within two days, the number of similar cases and deaths increased. On July 14, the test result from Sichuan Provincial CDC demonstrated a negative result for IgG, and IgM against hemorrhagic fever. At 12:00 pm on July 15, Ziyang Health Bureau reported to the Provincial Health Bureau (current Health and Family Planning Commission) by telephone that an unknown disease occurred in Ziyang, with a total of 5 cases, 4 of whom died, and serological results of 5 cases suggested that a negative result of IgM against hemorrhagic fever, and increase of urine protein. Severe cases presented with toxic shock symptoms and died.

On July 15, Sichuan Provincial Health Bureau convened experts in epidemiology, laboratory technicians from Provincial CDC and clinical experts from provincial hospital to investigate in Ziyang. The experts went to the hospital to learn the conditions of the patients and treatments, with clinical experts providing guidance on treatments in the hospital, and with experts from Provincial CDC collecting and testing blood samples again. Experts from Provincial CDC also went to the patients' families to investigate the surrounding environments, and suggested the disease was associated with (dead) pig, when they found a dead pig in a neighbor's house. They immediately collected samples from the dead pig and at the same time blood samples from the family members of patients for lab testing. However, the experts' opinions differed regarding the diagnosis after investigation and consultation: some experts suggested hemorrhagic fever with renal syndrome, and some experts suggested exclusion of hemorrhagic fever with renal syndrome due to the association with pigs and sheep. In the evening of July 15, Sichuan Provincial Health Bureau notified the outbreak to the emergency office of former Ministry of Health (current Emergency Office of Health and Family Planning Commission). At 0:45 of July 16, Yanjiang District CDC of Ziyang Prefecture reported the outbreak of an unknown disease through Information Management System of Public Health Emergency.

In the early stage of the investigation, based on the limited information, the case definition was: "cases with sudden fever accompanied with symptoms of septic shock such as ecchymosis and petechiae in skin, onset recently in Yanjiang district or adjacent rural areas, who had contacted with sick (dead) pigs (sheep)".

On July 18, the investigation team searched possible cases according to the above case definition in the Third People's Hospital of Ziyang, investigated in the patients 'neighbors' houses and found 7 cases with 5 dead. A case-based investigation was carried out to learn the basic characteristics of the outbreak.

The first patient: WU, male, 52 years old. He developed sudden fever (38.2℃), chills, nausea and vomiting, body pain, ecchymosis and other symptoms at 11:50 in the morning of June 24, and died on the way to hospital at 19:00. He contacted with the dead sheep owned by Peng (another case) at 11 am of June 22.

The onset date of the 7 patients was June 24, June 26, July 5, July 9, July 10, July 16, and July 17. The cases were distributed in 6 villages of 4 towns in 2 districts in Ziyang prefecture. There were 6 males and 1 female, who were all farmers. The time from onset to death for the 5 dead cases ranged from 4 hours to 21 hours with an average of 11.6 hours. There were pigs (sheep) which were sick (dead) in local rural before the onset of the 7 cases. Of the 7 patients, 5 slaughtered sick (dead) pigs/ sheep before onset, 2 participated in processing of sick (dead) pigs/sheep before onset. Incubation from recent slaughter or contact with sick (dead) pigs (sheep) to onset ranged from less than 1 day to 5 days. Broken skin with blackened wounds and few pus were observed in hand and arm in one case. No cases were observed among the other 6 people who were involved in the slaughtering. No cases were observed in 140 villagers who participated in cooking and eating the dead pig meat. No similar cases were observed among close contacts of the cases, including family members, neighbors, relatives, medical staff, and patients in the same wards. Of the 7 cases, except for Peng and Wu who contacted the same dead sheep, all others had a history of contact with a different sick (dead) pig.

"A strange disease struck". The news spread like wildfire, with widely spreading through the web and the media. The media were full of the words of "strange disease", and "unknown disease". The general people were still scared of the unknown disease because it was just a couple years after SARS in 2003-2004. The disease had an acute onset, progressed rapidly with high fatality, and the etiology was not identified. The panic spread in the crowd, so that the people resisted to eat pork and were afraid of even talking about the pig. The pork from Sichuan was banned and the purchased inventory was seized in some areas. Sichuan is a large Province with pig industry which was then severely affected. The outbreak in Ziyang occurred in pigs for retail in the rural area with poor farming conditions. There was no disease found in large scale pig farms. However, the small problem from an isolated area imposed an overall adverse impact on the whole industry. Affected by the outbreak, the local people didn't dare to purchase or eat pork; the price of pig and pork fell in some areas and sales decreased sharply; and some large livestock processing enterprises were influenced.

Preliminary investigation showed that the disease was highly sporadic, which was associated with the contact with sick/dead pigs. SARS and epidemic hemorrhagic fever with renal syndrome were excluded, although the etiology was still unknown. During outbreak and epidemic of infectious diseases, laboratory testing of pathogenic microorganisms is critical for confirmation of clinical cases, appropriate treatment, identification of the causes of outbreak, tracking the source of infection, cutting off the route of transmission, and providing important evidence for development of effective prevention and control measures. Lab results are also the key to eliminate the panic. Now all public attentions focused on CDC system which just experienced the SARS outbreak. It was time to test the capacity of CDC system.

5.2 Expert group sent by Ministry of Health

On July 18, 2005, China CDC received the report from Sichuan Provincial

CDC that an unknown disease occurred in the city of Ziyang with a total of 7 cases reported, including 5 deaths. Hemorrhagic fever with rena/symdrome was excluded, and the preliminary diagnosis was infectious sepsis. Bacterial infection was suspected due to high white blood cell counts. The cause of death was septic shock. After receiving the report, China CDC reported the outbreak quickly to Ministry of Health. Leadership from Ministry of Health attached great importance to the Sichuan's outbreak, both Minister Gao Qiang and Vice Minister Wang Longde gave important instructions. An expert team consisted of experts in epidemiology, clinical and laboratory was immediately sent to the site to help guide the response to the outbreak. In the evening of June 18, led by Yang Weizhong, Director of Office of Emergency, China CDC, the national expert team joined the local experts to set up a joint investigation team. In the afternoon of June 19, the team rushed to Ziyang City, with emergency leadership team being set up at front-line to guide responses to outbreak. In accordance with the principle of simultaneous investigation and response during public health emergency, a strategy was developed to treat the patients and at the same time to carry out on-site survey, to find out the cause as soon as possible, and to develop the control strategy. As to the pathogen, Streptococcus suis infection was highly suspected. Control measures included cutting off the transmission route from sick pig to human through slaughtering sick pigs.

In collaboration with local health departments and CDCs at all levels, the national and Provincial Working Group set up different teams for leadership, epidemiological investigation, laboratory testing, clinical treatment, pathology and logistics issues, with responsibilities and jobs clarified for each team. With professional teams established, the experts worked hard to implement the measures immediately. A series of protocols on disease prevention and control were developed; the patients were treated; the cases were searched; epidemiological survey was conducted on the source of infection, transmission route, high-risk (susceptible) population and risk factors; the samples were collected; laboratory pathogenic testing was carried out, including isolation by culture and molecular biological assay.

5.3 Extensive epidemiological investigation

On July 19, epidemiological investigation team urgently developed a standard form for epidemiological survey, and carried out the case-based investigation on July 20. According to the geographical distribution of cases, the epidemiological investigation team was further divided into 3 groups going to Yanjiang district and Jianyang City, to complete the investigation of all cases and matched controls, and to carry out active searching of cases according to the "case definition", standard method and procedure, so as to fully learn the situations of the outbreak. Afterwards, the investigation team went to the medical institutions, rural areas, farmers' families, to investigate the newly detected cases, suspected cases, and close contacts in accordance with the same methods and procedures. The data was entered into computer timely for epidemiological analysis. The outbreak information was summarized and reported daily to provide objective data timely for scientific decisions by leaders and experts at all levels. These data demonstrated the transmission route, and provided supporting data for identification of the cause of the disease.

During the searching, some cases presenting mainly with meningitis in rural areas had also a history of contact with sick (dead) pigs except for toxic shock syndrome. With the progress of the on-site investigation and pathogenic diagnosis, the understanding of the disease was deepened, and gradually the cases with manifestations of meningitis, mild cases with a contact history were included in the case definition. The case definition was updated as: cases presenting with acute fever, accompanied by petechiae and ecchymosis in skin, possibly complicated by meningitis or septic shock, etc.; onset since June in Yanjiang District and adjacent rural areas; contacts with sick (dead) pigs (sheep) before onset.

According to the new case definition, a total of 55 cases (majority were clinically diagnosed) were detected and investigated by the end of July 23, all of whom were local farmers, with more male than female. The age ranged from 32 to 75 years old, with an average of 51.6 years old. Most of the patients aged from 50 to 60 years old, accounting for about 32.7%. The first case occurred on June 24, and the incidence increased since early July with a peak on July 19.

Most patients presented with chills, fever, headache, dizziness, malaise, fatigue at early stage; some patients had nausea and vomiting and other gastrointestinal symptoms, and a minority of patients presented with abdominal pain and diarrhea. Severe cases manifested with septic shock with low BP, decreased SBP-DBP; most cases presented with petechiae and ecchymosis in skin; while some cases didn't manifest septic shock, but with positive meningeal signs and purulent cerebrospinal fluid. Coma was observed in severe cases. The organ damage was observed in severe patients, including interstitial pulmonary edema, liver damage and kidney damage. Laboratory results: elevated white blood cell (reduced or normal in early stage in severe cases), increased neutrophils and thrombocytopenia in severe cases. Urine protein was positive and acetone positive in some patients.

The analysis showed that 49 out of 55 cases had a history of suspected risk exposure, and the contact history for the other 6 cases was unknown. Among them, 47 cases contacted with dead pigs and 2 cases contacted with dead sheep. Contact types included feeding, slaughtering, selling, washing and cutting, eating, burying (dead) pigs (sheep). On average, the skin of the arm was broken or scratched in 37.2% cases when contacting. There were no other obvious common factors among the cases, such as exposure to animals, foods or water. No evidence of contacting among the cases, and no secondary cases were observed in close contacts and family members. The case-control study showed that slaughter, skin damage and bleeding wound were risk factors.

5.4   Treatment of severely ill patients and reducing fatality rate

To better treat the severely ills and reduce fatality rate, clinical team designated hospitals to admit and treat patients. Experts in infectious diseases and anti-shock from large hospitals in Beijing, Chengdu, Nanjing were invited to the designated hospitals and work with local doctors to treat patient as well as to train the local doctors. The experts went all out to treat the patients to minimize death rate.

5.5   The laboratory testing: final confirmation

The laboratory team overcame various difficulties to go to farmers' families, medical institutions, and funeral institutions to collect samples. The dead cases were autopsied, at the same time the dead or dying pigs were autopsied, with a large number of qualified samples collected. The samples were transported immediately to China CDC in Beijing. China CDC, Sichuan Provincial CDC and some hospitals simultaneously conducted the lab testing. Laboratory staff worked round the clock to culture the bacteria and identify the microorganisms using ATB and PCR. On July 23, Streptococcus suis serotype 2 was detected from the patient's blood, spleen samples and dead pig organ samples. Lab results showed that these strains were compatible to Streptococcus suis serotype 2 in morphology, biochemical reaction and virulent genes Figure 5.2. There are in total 35 serotypes of Streptococcus suis, with serotype 2 the most common in human infection. All the isolates from humans and pigs have all the virulent genes of Streptococcus suis. The 7 specific genes of the three strains were amplified or cloned by staff of State Key Laboratory of Infectious Disease Prevention and Control in Institute of Infectious Disease Prevention and Control, led by Xu Jianguo. The sequencing conducted by State Key Laboratory of Virus Gene Engineering was fully compatible with the sequence of Streptococcus suis published, and the sequences of strains from pig and human were the same.

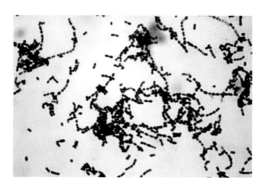

Figure 5.2   Streptococcus suis, Gram stain (Source: multimedia of Merck Veterinary).

5.6 Determination of the cause of outbreak as Streptococcus suis, and release to the public

According to clinical presentation, epidemiological investigation and laboratory results, it was confirmed that the outbreak was caused by Streptococcus suis, with the main rationale as follows:

- Incubation period, the main clinical symptoms, signs and laboratory results were compatible with the published infections with Streptococcus suis (common type, toxic shock syndrome type and meningitis type).
- History of exposure to dead pigs before onset, and no secondary cases and no other common exposure, such as animals, foods or water, all provided supporting evidence.
- Outbreaks of Streptococcus suis infection in local swine herd occurred.
- Identification of Streptococcus suis isolated from blood and spleen samples of 3 patients were compatible with Streptococcus suis serotype 2 in morphology, biochemical reaction, and Streptococcus suis specific virulent gene. Streptococcus suis were also isolated from the pig which was contacted by 2 cases before onset, and from local sick (dead) pigs.

On July 25, Ministry of Health and Ministry of Agriculture jointly released the news to the public, that the outbreak was human infections with Streptococcus suis.

Streptococcus is a gram positive cocci, which is divided into 20 serogroups according to serological reaction. Different serogroup is specific to different animal hosts in pathogenicity. Some serogroups could cause disease in pigs, and some serogroups, such as R, F group, could cause disease in both pigs and humans. Human infection with Streptococcus suis and resulting in disease is relatively rare, which was first described by Danish scholar in 1968 with meningitis caused by human infection of Streptococcus suis. Some human infection with type II of R group Streptococcus suis were reported abroad in recent years, but with few cases (on average 1 - 2 cases) per event. Streptococcus suis outbreak was reported in 1998 in Nantong, Jiangsu Province in China. Human infection with Streptococcus suis serotype 2 is usually associated with purulent meningitis, deafness, movement disorders, and toxic shock syndrome, multiple organ failure and death in severe cases. Human infection with Streptococcus suis generally occurs among the butchers, animal farm workers, staff in raw meat processing and sales, and occasionally among poachers of wild boar. A history of close contact with pigs and pork are all reported before onset, therefore, some scholars think that human infection with Streptococcus suis is an occupational zoonosis.

Since understanding of Streptococcus suis is inadequate and the morphological and biochemical features of Streptococcus suis is easy to change, its isolation and identification is difficult. Clinicians do not know much about the disease, and the hospital and CDC at grassroots level don't have the capacity to detect the pathogen. Based on experience and lessons learnt from SARS, the capacity of public health system in China had been strengthened to respond to public health emergencies, and to isolate and identify pathogenic microorganisms. China CDC supplemented a few laboratory kits of newly emergent, imported and rare infectious diseases and technical capacity. This is the key to detect the pathogen and to identify the nature of the outbreak. Chinese CDC system provided a satisfactory answer in this outbreak.

5.7 Implementation of measures to control the outbreak

At the same time of investigation, the control measures were implemented. The investigation provided breakthrough progress so that the joint expert group modified and improved the case definition and treatment protocol again. "Diagnostic Criteria of Streptococcus Suis Infection in Humans in Sichuan Provine", "Treatment Protocol of Humans Infection with Streptococcus Suis in Sichuan Province (Trial)" and "Technical Standard for Prevention and Control of Streptococcus Suis" were developed to provide recommendations and scientific strategies on prevention and control of the disease timely for local government. The local government was responsible for the organization, supervision and logistics support to ensure the implementation of prevention and control measures.

The comprehensive measures of prevention and control of human infection with Streptococcus suis is presented in Figure 5.3.

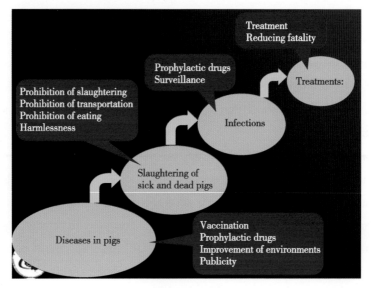

Figure 5.3　Comprehensive strategies for prevention and control of Streptococcus suis.

5.7.1　Implementation of monitoring and reporting, improvement of capacity to early signal detection of, and early response to outbreak

First, various technical programs were developed and revised timely to guide the scientific prevention and control of the outbreak. For example, epidemiological investigation program of human infection with Streptococcus suis, case reporting procedure, outbreak verification procedure, and "Program of Epidemiological Investigation and Surveillance of Human Infection with Streptococcus Suis Serotype 2" were developed, so as to standardize the criteria for surveillance and clinical diagnosis. Second, all social forces were mobilized; professional institutions and personnel were fully utilized to carry out an intensive outbreak census to timely detect and treat outbreak in human and animals. Since July 20, surveillance and case notification was gradually carried out in Sichuan Province, with all cases meeting the "case definition" at corresponding stage reported and with the cerebrospinal fluid and blood samples collected for pathogen isolation.

5.7.2　The spread of the disease was interrupted by utilizing the legal, administrative and technical strategies and approaches.

On one hand, in accordance with the *"Law on Prevention and Control of Infectious*

Disease", "Law on Prevention of Epidemic in Animal", "National Preparedness on Major Emergent Epidemic in Animal" and *"National Preparedness on Response to Public Health Emergency",* emergency response mechanism was timely initiated. On the other hand, the key measures of prevention and control were carried out fully to block the spread of disease. Expert group together with the local government carried out the new strategies named *"Five Contracts, Four Nos, Two Subsidies and One Harmlessness"* to block the transmission. "Five Contracts" means Prefecture contracting with County, County contracting with Township, Township contracting with village, and village contracting with group, group contracting with households, to clarify the responsibility of individual so as to block the spread of disease. "Four Nos" means no slaughtering, no eating, no selling, and no transportation of sick (dead) pigs outside. "Two subsidies" means subsidies for farmers to handle the sick (dead) pigs harmlessly and subsidies for treatment of the disease. "One harmlessness" means harmlessly handle the sick (dead) pigs with disinfection followed by deep burying by bleaching powder and quicklime or incineration. All above measures facilitated the blocking of the transmission route, containing of the outbreak, and preventing the spreading to human being.

In order to prevent the dead pigs entering into the market, Ziyang Prefecture set up 24 temporary quarantine sites in the major roads, and 117 mobile inspection sites in foci areas. At the same time, a census of dead pigs of unknown causes was carried out. The census found about 400 dead pigs of unknown causes which were harmlessly handled.

The government promptly issued economic compensation policies, which effectively promoted the harmless handling of sick (dead) pigs. On July 17, expert group of Sichuan Provincial Health Bureau recommended to the local health administrative departments to discourage and prohibit farmers from slaughtering and eating sick (dead) pigs. However, these recommendations were not implemented so that the cases continued to increase.

On July 19, the national and provincial joint expert group discussed with Ziyang government on prevention and control of the outbreak, stressing the importance of discouraging and prohibiting farmers from slaughtering and eating sick (dead) pigs. The government believed that publicity and education should be combined with

prevention of summer diseases in order to avoid the influence on economic development and social stability by excessive public opinions, and to avoid social panic due
to excessive publicity. Eventually, the government tried to alert the public by the
announcement: to reduce the contact with sick (dead) pigs. However, for the poor
farmers, pigs are an important source of income, so that slaughtering and eating sick
(dead) pigs still persisted in rural areas, and cases continued to increase.

On July 22, new cases continued to occur in the surrounding counties and
cities. Ministry of Health released the news of the outbreak through the media in the
evening of July 22 for the first time. Considering that the disease was prevalent in
animals, it was difficult to control the outbreak in human. Therefore, the government
modified the strategy to require that "slaughtering sick (dead) pigs is prohibited" in
the form of government order, and the families with sick (dead) pigs were compen-
sated economically; and township (town) officials were required to be responsible
for the implementation of "prohibition of slaughtering" by contracting with villages,
publicity and education and harmless handling of sick (dead) pigs. Afterwards,
the effectiveness of control measures was demonstrated, with the number of cases
decreasing rapidly (Figure 5.4).

5.7.3 Enhancement of the prevention and control of epidemic in animals.

Firstly, the sensitive prophylactic antibiotics was administered to the pigs in the
same pig pens with the sick pig; secondly, the farmers were instructed to add prophylactic antibiotics in the feed to improve immunity; thirdly, the pig pens, trading
places, slaughtering sites were disinfected regularly in the affecting areas to improve
hygiene conditions; lastly, the emergency immunization in pigs was carried out to
improve the herd immunity. As of August 20, 9.923 million pigs were provided the
immunization from 2.978 million farmers in 1569 townships in the affected areas in
Ziyang with a coverage rate of 73%.

5.7.4 Strengthening publicity and risk communication, elimination of social panic and mobilization of public to cooperate

The information of the outbreak was transparent, timely released to the public, and notified to WHO and Hongkong, Macao Special Administrative Regions. Publicity of prevention and control of Streptococcus suis was strengthened in all areas. Meanwhile, under cooperation with the media, publicity regarding transmission route, clinical symptoms and prevention measures of Streptococcus suis serotype 2 was carried out. Efforts were made to ensure that all farmers implemented the measures of prevention and control, and all farmers received the knowledge of prevention and control, so as to increase the awareness of raising pigs in a scientific way and of disease prevention. Health education was carried out locally in the popular form, with difficult words avoided and easily understandable words used, for example, "no transportation and processing sick/dead pigs" was modified to "no carrying, no washing and cutting sick/dead pigs".

In the evening of July 22, the news of Streptococcus suis was released for the first time, which resulted in great concern in social media at first. The Ministry of Health updated the cases and deaths by news daily, but did not release the cause, risk factors, or measures of prevention and control at the early stage. Therefore, some media began to use attractive words such as "Sichuan disease" and "unexplained disease". Some media even used the word of "deadly pork" for the source of infection. Due to the inadequate guidance on publicity, people in Sichuan Province were panic about "pig" and refused to buy or eat any pork or pork products. During that time, local government officials were in conflict with reporters due to media reports on the outbreak. After the media reported the outbreak in Sichuan Province, active surveillance and retrospective searching of cases were carried out in Sichuan Province to detect lots of sporadic cases in multiple areas with reported infections of Streptococcus suis increasing, which caused more social and public panic. Some Provincial (municipal) governments even issued an order to ban all importation of pig, pork and pork products from Sichuan.

On July 26, with the pathogen confirmed, the news office of Ministry of Health formally reported the outbreak of "human infection with Streptococcus suis", and thereafter media reports became accurate and standard, which facilitated the formulation of correct attitudes of the public to the outbreak and to the contact with sick/ dead pig (sheep).

The government of Sichuan Province issued a series of orders which prohibited the slaughtering of sick/dead pigs which should be handled harmlessly (disinfection followed by deep-bury or incineration). Thus, the route of transmission was blocked, and the outbreak was completely controlled. The temporal distribution of cases is shown in figure 5.4.

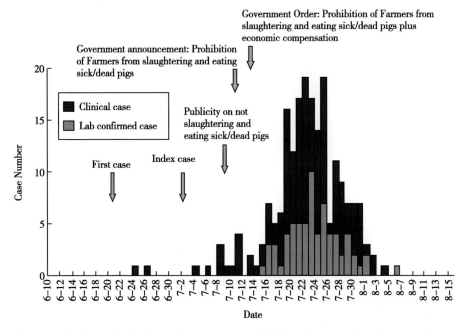

Figure 5.4   Time distribution of human cases with Streptococcus Suis by onset time.

5.8 Control of the outbreak with remarkable impacts

Since the outbreak of SARS, CDCs in China has improved the capacity to respond to emergent acute infectious disease and passed the test of "strange disease" by identifying the cause of and controlling the outbreak successfully.

On August 21, 2005, the Ministry of Health and the Ministry of Agriculture jointly issued the "Evaluation report of the outbreak of Streptococcus Suis in Sichuan Province" which confirmed the pathogen and transmission route of the outbreak in late June in some areas of Sichuan Province after the investigation and joint efforts by the Sichuan Government, the Ministry of Health and the Ministry of Agriculture. The measures of prevention and control were fully carried out; the medical treatment was effective; and obvious achievements were made in terms of prevention and control. With comprehensive evaluation by the experts, it was concluded that the outbreak of Streptococcus Suis in Sichuan Province had been controlled effectively.

The evaluation report pointed out that, according to the laboratory and epidemiological findings, the outbreak in Sichuan Province was caused by Streptococcus suis serotype 2. The cases were concentrated in some isolated areas of Sichuan, mainly in remote and poor rural areas. Streptococcus suis disease in pigs is categorized as a type 2 animal disease in China, which mainly infects pigs in the backyard breeding sites with poor sanitation, poor ventilation and damp pens. The pigs in the same pen are not likely to be infected. In general, large farms and large-scale farm industry with good sanitary conditions are relatively less influenced by the outbreak. Human infection with Streptococcus Suis were all caused by secret slaughtering and processing the sick/dead pigs. There is no interpersonal transmission of the disease and no one was infected due to purchasing or eating pork which was adequately quarantined.

After the outbreak, the CPC Central Committee and State Council attached great importance. CPC and governments at all levels in Sichuan Province took action quickly, to study and carry out the prevention and control measures, and to initiate the emergency response. A series of effective measures were implemented according to the emergency response plan, with epidemiological investigation undertaken, sick/dead pigs and related products managed strictly, patients treated actively, knowledge of disease prevention delivered, supervision and inspection strengthened. The Ministry of Health closely cooperated with the Ministry of Agriculture and other Ministries, to establish the temporary working group for prevention and control of Streptococcus Suis. Ministers of the two Ministries went to the affected areas and sent supervision team and expert team to guide and support local investigation and handling of the outbreak, to implement the measures of prevention and control and to treat patients. Meanwhile, the outbreak information was released to the public in a timely manner and was notified to Hongkong and Macao Special Administrative Regions and to WHO and other international organizations.

In total, 204 cases were found during the outbreak in Sichuan, of whom 68 were pathogenically confirmed (isolation of Streptococcus Suis serotype 2). Among the confirmed cases, 38 were confirmed by blood samples, 27 by cerebrospinal fluid and 3 by autopsy samples (liver, spleen, heart blood). The confirmed cases were distributed in 11 cities in Sichuan Province, and the same pathogens were isolated from pigs in different areas.

References

1. Yang Weizhong, Yu Hongjie, Jing Huaiqi, et al. An outbreak of Human infection with Streptococcus Suis serotype 2 accompanied by toxic shock syndrome in Sichuan Provincial. Chinese Journal of epidemiology, 2006; 27 (3): 185-191.

2. Yu H, Jing H, Chen Z, Zheng H, Zhu X, et al. Human Streptococcus suis outbreak, Sichuan, China. Emerg Infect Dis,2006; 12:914-12:9

3. Yu Hongjie, Liu Xuecheng, Wang Shiwen, et al. A Matched case-control study of risk factors of Streptococcus suis infection in Sichuan Provincial. The Chinese Journal of epidemiology, 2005; 26 (9): 636-639.

4. Wang Longde. Case study and analysis of field epidemiology. Beijing: People's Medical Publishing House, 2006.

图书在版编目（CIP）数据

中国公共卫生. 重大疾病防治实践 = Infectious
Disease in China：the Best Practical Cases：英文 /
杨维中主编. —北京：人民卫生出版社，2018
　　ISBN 978-7-117-26001-5

　Ⅰ．①中…　Ⅱ．①杨…　Ⅲ．①公共卫生－中国－英文
②疾病－防治－中国－英文　Ⅳ．①R1②R4

中国版本图书馆 CIP 数据核字（2018）第 133197 号

人卫智网	www.ipmph.com	医学教育、学术、考试、健康，
		购书智慧智能综合服务平台
人卫官网	www.pmph.com	人卫官方资讯发布平台

中国公共卫生：重大疾病防治实践（英文）

主　　编：杨维中
出版发行：人民卫生出版社（中继线 010-59780011）
地　　址：北京市朝阳区潘家园南里 19 号
邮　　编：100021
E - mail：pmph @ pmph.com
购书热线：010-59787592　　010-59787584　　010-65264830
印　　刷：北京盛通印刷股份有限公司
经　　销：新华书店
开　　本：710×1000　1/16　　**印张：**7
字　　数：122 千字
版　　次：2018 年 11 月第 1 版　2018 年 11 月第 1 版第 1 次印刷
标准书号：ISBN 978-7-117-26001-5
打击盗版举报电话：010-59787491　　E-mail：WQ @ pmph.com
（凡属印装质量问题请与本社市场营销中心联系退换）